✔ KU-534-884

TIMELESS HEALING

THE POWER AND BIOLOGY OF BELIEF

HERBERT BENSON, MD
WITH MARG STARK

POCKET
BOOKS

LONDON · SYDNEY · NEW YORK · TOKYO · SINGAPORE · TORONTO

First published in Great Britain by Simon & Schuster Ltd, 1996

First published in paperback by Pocket Books, 1998
An imprint of Simon & Schuster Ltd
A Viacom company

1 3 5 7 9 10 8 6 4 2

Simon & Schuster Ltd
West Garden Place
Kendal Street
London W2 2AQ

Simon & Schuster Australia
Sydney

A CIP catalogue record for this book is available from the British
Library

ISBN 0-67185520-4

To life!

ACKNOWLEDGMENTS

I gratefully acknowledge my colleagues at the Mind/Body Medical Institute, the Deaconess Hospital, and the Harvard Medical School, without whose many contributions to the field of mind/body medicine this work would not have been possible. Whenever I could, I have tried to mention their names in the text.

Over my thirty years at Harvard Medical School, many different institutions, corporations, and foundations have supported my research and teaching activities with their financial contributions. My thanks to all of them for enabling me to present the theories of this book. Current funding sources for Mind/Body Medical Institute projects include: The California Wellness Foundation; The John Templeton Foundation; Sam Wyly Fund of the Communities Foundation of Texas, Inc.; Charles J. Wyly Fund of the Communities Foundation of Texas, Inc.; Castle Rock Foundation; William K. Coors; David B. Kriser; State Street Foundation; Amelior Foundation; Lewis N. Madeira; The Charles Englehard Foundation; Laurance S. Rockefeller; The Masco Foundation; and The Harold Grinspoon Charitable Foundation. The Trustees of the Mind/Body Medical Institute have been an unstinting reservoir of support whose friendship, time, talent, and financial contributions have ensured the growth and successful future of the Institute.

For her expertise in helping with the book's references, I am most grateful to Patricia Zuttermeister. For his wise counsel, I wish to thank my attorney, Robert E. Cowden III. I also thank Arrco Medical Art and Design, Inc., for their fine artwork.

This work evolved with the expert creative advice of my literary agent, Patti Breitman. I wish to thank her for her insight, which graced the project from start to finish. I am grateful also to publisher Susan Moldow for her commitment to the work and for her editorial contributions.

I was so impressed with Marg Stark when she interviewed me for a magazine article on unconventional medicine that I asked her to be my collaborator on this book. Our subsequent friendship has been a joy. Her writing skills and original contributions have made my choice inspired.

On her behalf, Marg Stark has asked me to acknowledge Dennis Hawk for his legal counsel. She also wishes to thank her parents, Bill and Joyce, for living their beliefs, and her husband, Darwin, for believing in her.

The individual contributions of patients are often lost in the conclusions of scientific data. Ultimately though, individuals who agreed to participate in studies made the research findings of this book possible. I am grateful to them, as I am to my patients who shared their stories in this book.

Finally, I am forever grateful to my wife, Marilyn, for her unending support and advice.

CONTENTS

FOREWORD

In my previous books, I have focused on the things that individuals can do to heal themselves. As I tracked modes of self-care, trying to "isolate" benefits and "reduce" these therapies to their purest forms, a much larger principle emerged. I became impressed with the human trait to turn to beliefs and faith in times of illness and need, and so I spent more than thirty years developing the findings I present in this book. Practicing medicine and conducting medical research, I've learned that invoking beliefs is not only emotionally and spiritually soothing but vitally important to physical health.

I have had the privilege of observing belief-inspired healing in many of my patients. But to enable them to speak freely about their experiences with "remembered wellness" and "the faith factor," I asked my collaborator Marg Stark to interview them and to recount their histories. I also ensured confidentiality by changing their names even though virtually all of them granted permission to use their true names.

I have also chosen to fully reference the scientific documentations of the book. So at the end you will find an extensive list of the scientific articles and books published on these subjects. It is my hope that this kind of evidence will form a platform upon which my scientific colleagues will further build. Perhaps then remembered wellness and the faith factor will be better recognized and implemented in medical practice.

This book is written to help people help themselves. Should you choose to apply these teachings to your medical therapy, do so in partnership with a physician to take full advantage of the solutions and cures conventional medicine has to offer.

The biology of belief ensures that it is ever present in medicine and health of all kinds whether or not its effects are acknowledged. Timelessly influential, our values and life experiences cannot help but manifest themselves. My hope is that this book will help you appreciate the power of your beliefs so you can embrace life, and the meaning of your life, for the fullest measure of health.

HERBERT BENSON, MD
Boston, Massachusetts

CHAPTER 1

A SEARCH FOR SOMETHING THAT LASTS

When I was a student at Harvard Medical School, I was taught that the greater part of what I was learning about the human body would be obsolete within five years. In other words, a few years after I finished medical school, before I even completed my hospital residency and became a full-fledged member of the medical profession, medical science would have progressed so far as to create a whole new set of rules for taking care of patients.

Thus began my search for something in medicine that lasts. I wanted to identify some timeless source of healing, the merits of which could never be denied. Not only would this "treatment of choice" outlast the five-year mark but it would have proven value for generations present, for generations past, and for generations to come.

I will confess that, in part, youthful laziness launched my search. No medical student relishes the idea of having to learn a subject over and over again. But my contemplation of the enduring aspects of human life began in earnest when I was twenty-one, a premed student in college, and had to face the death of my father from rheumatic heart disease. In my mind, science never adequately explained his passing. With their diagrams, definitions, and anatomic drawings, my textbooks couldn't begin to capture the spirit and presence he embodied.

This was a man who had grown up in the jungles of South America, who came to the United States with only a fourth-grade education, who spoke five languages, and who went on to become a successful businessman in the wholesale and retail produce industry in Yonkers, New York. My father tried to impress upon me and my siblings the importance of "doing things right." He told us about the time a shopkeeper had had to let him go from his job sweeping up. To finish the job well, my dad was especially thorough cleaning up that night, so the next day the shopkeeper called to tell my father that if he was willing to return, the shopkeeper would find the financial means to keep him on.

This was what defined my father's life, the same way that

family and work, hardships and victories, principles and life lessons define the lives of all human beings. But these matters were rarely addressed in the education I received as a physician—in the scientific literature, in grand rounds, or even in the training I received at the bedside. And as much as I began to believe that science was all-powerful, snowballing in its ability to track and explain life's mysteries, I had a nagging feeling that medicine was missing a critical point.

Accumulating the Evidence

This book traces my steps over thirty years of accumulating evidence of an eternal truth about human physiology and the human experience. Luck, hunches, and happenstance often guided my journey, as with most people's careers. I went from patient to patient, from research study to research study in the same way that all physician-researchers do, unable to predict how each line of inquiry and its corresponding results would contribute to long-term improvements in medicine. But deep down, I always hoped that some immutable wisdom would emerge.

Partly because my father had died from heart disease, I started my career as a cardiologist. But soon I began to feel inhibited by my specialty, which limited its explorations to keeping chambered organs pumping in patients' chests. Increasingly, I was drawn to mind/body research, and would go on to become one of a handful of medical investigators who established the scientific field recognized today as mind/body medicine.

Except for a brief training stint in Seattle, and the time I spent in the U.S. Public Health Service in San Juan, Puerto Rico, I've spent my entire career working within Harvard Medical School's teaching hospitals. In 1988, I founded Harvard's Mind/Body Medical Institute at Boston's Deaconess Hospital. Perhaps my most significant contribution to the field was in defining a bodily calm that all of us can evoke and that has the opposite effect of the well-known fight-or-flight response. I call this bodily calm "the relaxation response," a state in which blood pressure is lowered, and heart rate, breathing rate, and metabolic rate are decreased. The relaxation response yields many long-term benefits in both health and well-being and can be brought on with very simple mental focusing or meditation techniques.

Teaching these methods to patients, health care professionals, and others, I began to realize the power of self-care, the healthy things that individuals can do for themselves. More and more, I became convinced that our bodies are wired to benefit from exercising not only our muscles but our rich inner, human core—our beliefs, values, thoughts, and feelings. I was reluctant to explore these factors because philosophers and scientists have, through the ages, considered them intangible and unmeasurable, making any study of them "unscientific." But I wanted to try, because, again and again, my patients' progress and recoveries often seemed to hinge upon their spirit and will to live. And I could not shake the sense I had that the human mind—and the beliefs we so often associate with the human soul—had physical manifestations.

First Hints of Mind/Body Influence

I had witnessed this firsthand while serving as a merchant seaman the summer after my junior year of college. From the time I read Joseph Conrad as a youth, I was determined to "go to sea." And together with my best friend Howard Rotner, I fulfilled this dream by acquiring this incredible "summer job," which took me across oceans and to ports as diverse as Casablanca, Morocco; Naples, Italy; Piraeus, Greece; Southampton, England; Istanbul and Izmir, Turkey. In these ports, my fellow seamen were fond of barroom bingeing and often returned to the ship with awful hangovers. Knowing that I planned to be a doctor, my suffering shipmates would come to me for relief. But all I had to offer them were vitamins, which I promptly dispensed.

Though the vitamins should have had little or no effect, my shipmates' symptoms—and foul moods—improved rapidly and dramatically after taking the pills. And as word spread of the wondrous results, more and more of my fellow sailors sought me out for my magic pills. But once my indoctrination into medicine began, I found my medical mentors and peers far less interested in this phenomenon. For the first time, I realized there was a great disparity between the things laypeople *felt* were good for them and those that medical scientists decided *were* good for them.

This disparity made me uncomfortable, as did the fact that a diagnosis—a few words from a doctor—could dramatically change a patient's view of him- or herself. On the basis of an office visit and a simple test, a doctor could, for example, in diagnosing hypertension, ask a patient to take medication for the rest of his or her life, to endure aggravating side effects, and make major adjustments in diet and lifestyle. Overnight, patients diagnosed with chronic medical problems or illnesses began to think of themselves as "sick," and the effect that label had on their psyches and their physical health was substantial.

This is what happened to a patient of mine, Antonia Baquero. Before I met her, Ms. Baquero had had calcium deposits removed from her breast, an operation that left a large indentation. The calcium deposits were benign, but her surgeon recommended the operation because of the relatively small chance that a malignant tumor might later develop. The mere suggestion that she might develop cancer frightened Ms. Baquero. "I panicked," she explains. "I decided immediately, in one moment, to have the calcium deposits removed." Later, she regretted the decision. "My body felt cut up. It was a very difficult time in my life. I was trying to juggle business and family. I would wake up at three A.M. and be unable to sleep. There was too much tension."

Seeking relief from the anxiety and panic that escalated after her surgery, Ms. Baquero happened to pick up my book *Your Maximum Mind* at the library. Soon after, she came to Boston from her home in New York to see me. I talked with her about the relaxation response and the ways in which this relaxed physical condition could be brought about, or "elicited" as I prefer to say. To elicit the response, I explained that she needed to focus silently on a word or phrase for a period of ten to twenty minutes twice every day, gently brushing aside any everyday thoughts that distracted her to return to her focus. I told her that this was the mental exercise I had shown would dramatically ease the body's usual alert mode of operation, not undermining it, simply letting it calm down and rest for a while while one was awake.

As so many of my patients do, Ms. Baquero decided to incorporate a religious phrase in this mental focusing exercise. Since I encourage people to pick a focus that pleases them, she adopted a Spanish blessing, *"Jesu Christo ayudame, ampárame y curame,"* which means "Jesus Christ, help me, protect me, and cure me." Her mother said a similar blessing to her and her siblings as children before they left for school each day. And over the course of months in which she used this familiar prayer to elicit the relaxation response, Ms. Baquero began to feel liberated from the worry and strain that had bothered her incessantly before. "I started to feel better. I started looking at people and life in a different way. I put less pressure on myself," she says.

Surely, Ms. Baquero was experiencing the wonderful physical solace of the relaxation response, the opposite effect of the edgy, adrenaline rush we experience in the stress-induced fight-or-flight response. But she also spoke of a more emotional comfort, which the symbolism and meaning of her mother's blessing inspired. The emotional and spiritual balm seemed to affect her as much as the chemical and physical changes that occur during the relaxation response.

Not only was her body soothing itself but Ms. Baquero seemed to be reclaiming her identity—the essence of which was called into question when the threat of cancer was introduced to her. Each time she invoked this powerful prayer, she recalled her mother's faith in God's protection, and the faith instilled in her as a child. By introducing this tender comfort into her daily experience, she began to regain confidence both in her body and in herself to face the twists and turns of life.

Maybe Ms. Baquero's surgeon didn't know that the simple, preventive act of surgery he suggested would cause her so much long-term distress. In our society, doctors often prefer—and presume that patients want—to "do something" and "act" to treat or prevent illness or injury. But in Ms. Baquero's case, the diagnosis and the act of "doing something" undermined her faith in the strength of her body. Eliciting the relaxation response with her prayer, she regained a mental equilibrium and undoubtedly helped to ward off disease by doing something to calm her body and her fears.

Remembered Wellness

I learned a lot from these two observations of simple human healing. It turns out that by tracking the contribution a person's desire for health had on his or her health, and by cherishing the right of the individual to choose his or her own outlook, I found the clues of a scientifically profound source of healing. I call this source "remembered wellness." Like my shipmates, all of us project our intense desire for wellness onto the medicine we take. And like Ms. Baquero, all of us have the ability to "remember" the calm and confidence associated with health and happiness, but not just in an emotional or psychologically soothing way. This memory is also physical.

Remembered wellness isn't particularly mysterious. The evidence of its substantial, positive influence over the body has existed for centuries. It's known in the scientific community as "the placebo effect." But I hope to replace the term with "remembered wellness" not only because it more accurately describes the brain mechanics involved but because "the placebo effect" has become pejorative in medical usage. Members of the medical community often refer to its successes as "just the placebo effect" in much the same way as we tend to dismiss ailments as being "all in your head."

Most of us think of a placebo as a sugar pill, which, when dispensed by a physician, plays a kind of trick on a patient's mind, producing benefits for the body. And we know that researchers often rely on placebos—inert substances or procedures—to contrast results between a control group and those receiving an experimental therapy. But perhaps less well promoted is that an individual's belief empowers the placebo. The fact that the patient, caregiver, or both of them believe in the treatment contributes to better outcomes. Depending on the condition, sometimes affirmative beliefs are all we really need to heal us. Other times we need the collective force of our beliefs and appropriate medical interventions.

Yet, despite the fact that physicians have always acknowledged this phenomenon, we haven't heralded its efficacy or explored its therapeutic applications. As the ultimate insult, a placebo has often been called a "dummy pill." But the human body, with its propensity to turn a person's beliefs into a physical instruction, is not dumb. I first began reviewing the scientific literature on the placebo effect in the mid-1970s, and shortly thereafter began publishing and speaking on its potential therapeutic benefits. Together with colleagues, I found that in the patient cases we reviewed, the effect I call remembered wellness was 70 to 90 percent effective, doubling and tripling the success rate that had always been attributed to the placebo effect.

As my research has progressed, I have learned that as long as humans have roamed the earth, we have entertained beliefs. We have always called upon God or gods to sustain us. We have named and given meaning to nearly everything, sometimes simply in our own quiet contemplation of life, sometimes on a larger scale to stir the thoughts of whole populations, as happens in art, literature, and philosophy. We see the world in the unique way our socialization, life experiences, and cultural and religious upbringing permit us to see it. We are not all equally analytical or compelled to find deep meaning in the events of our lives, but we human beings cannot help but color our reality with hopes, emotions, philosophies, and convictions. It is our nature.

But neurological research reveals that before we consciously color the world around us with our thinking and acquired beliefs, brain mechanisms mark our perceptions, forming opinions and assigning emotional values. Before we even have a chance to mull over the presence of a new sight or sound, regions of our brain react by assigning an initial but influential value to it. These automatic attitudes make us incapable of utter objectivity or neutrality, in more profound ways than we've ever suspected.

Western science and all of its brilliant discoveries have been built on the tenet that we can and should want to achieve objectivity, and that objective facts can be distinguished from intangible or subjective aspects of life. And because beliefs and emotions are ephemeral and imperceptible, Western medicine has largely assumed that their effects are not physical or measurable. But neurological researchers and those of us delving into the considerable, measurable effects that beliefs can have on the human body are painting a very different portrait of human physiology and human life, with discoveries destined to change the way health care is conducted.

A Book About Beliefs

I could not have predicted that I would write an entire book about the fact that beliefs have physical repercussions, or that the human spirit was relevant, much less that it was influential, in the treatment and prevention of illnesses. But in my thirty years of practicing medicine, I've found no healing force more impressive or more universally accessible than the power of the individual to care for and cure him- or herself. But different from the message often championed in the public realm, it isn't belief in one's self, or a simple matter of positive thinking, that reaps the greatest health rewards. Nor is it as simple as turning away from Western medicine to rely on unconventional healers and their seemingly more sensitive healing arts.

I believe the ideal model for medicine is that of the three-legged stool (see Figure 1). The stool is balanced by the appropriate application of self-care, medications, and medical procedures. One leg, that which patients can do for themselves, is the most disparaged and neglected aspect of health care today. The other two legs are things the health care profession can offer or do for patients—resources that medicine relies on almost exclusively today, and that are splendid for the problems they actually solve. In this book, we'll focus on remembered wellness, which can enhance all three legs of the stool. Doctors and other caregivers dispensing medication or performing procedures must believe in their efficacy and communicate this confidence to patients to engender remembered wellness. But we'll pay special attention to the self-care leg of the stool, not so much on physical exercise and nutrition, which we all know are good for us, but on the inner development of beliefs that promote healing.

I'll lead you through the hypotheses and findings that propelled my process of discovery and show why we need greater balance among the three legs of the stool. Throughout my search and in this book, I have applied objective measurements to prove very subjective points, and used empirical data to draw conclusions about "intangibles"—about people's expectations, hopes, and fears. That these findings say so much about us as emotional, spiritual, and intellectual beings, and not just about our physicality and health, is a strange and wonderful by-product of a traditional scientific pursuit.

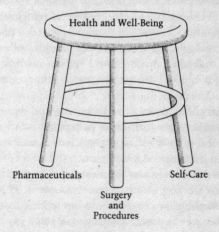

FIGURE 1

THE THREE-LEGGED STOOL

Health and well-being can be maximized with the balanced application of pharmaceuticals, surgery and procedures, and self-care. In medical practice today, the stool is unbalanced because we rely far too much on pharmaceuticals and surgery and procedures. We must embrace self-care to optimize medicine, health, and well-being as well as to balance the stool.

But my search also exposed the inherent weaknesses in Western thought and medicine, which has failed to appreciate the consistent power of remembered wellness. It's uncanny that medical science, in its passion to preserve life, has neglected the motivations that drive humankind forward, the meaning of life that makes people thirst for health and longevity.

There's a great deal of practical advice to come in this book that pays attention to these primal instincts. We'll explore the role beliefs play in your health and well-being, and strategies you can employ to "remember" wellness. We'll talk about the impact remembered wellness can have on medical conditions and illnesses, and suggest more appropriate use of medications and medical procedures for problems that cannot be solved by remembered wellness alone. Then I'll make recommendations about how to choose healthily from a menu of self-care, conventional, and unconventional healing options.

I'll conclude with a blueprint for optimal medicine and health that I believe takes full advantage of remembered wellness and the visceral nature of human beliefs. But when mobilized, the wisdom inherent in our bodies will not only transform individual health, it will reform medicine, saving our nation billions of dollars per year in unnecessary health care expenditures.

Many years have passed since I was a medical student, eager to use the science I was learning to help patients. Since then, as the pages of this book will describe, I have found a source of healing that is timeless. A basic instinct, this belief often transports people from pain and illness and, yet, to our detriment, Western science and society often dismisses it. This visceral truth is something we can count on, something that remains the same despite the dramatic changes we often experience in our public and private lives. We don't acquire it from textbooks; it is part of our physical endowment from the day we are born. This was true of my father and all the generations before him, it is true of you and your family, and it will be true of all our descendants. Eternally and internally true, it is an entrenched fact of human life that, when exercised and appreciated, has enormous power to heal us—mind, body, and soul.

CHAPTER 2

REMEMBERED
WELLNESS

Y ou make an appointment to see your doctor after a week or two of grappling with what feels like the world's worst respiratory infection. But by the time you get to the doctor's office, your symptoms have all but disappeared. You sit in the waiting room trying to conjure the fever, the chest-rattling cough, or at least a sniffle to dignify the pleas for mercy you made to the appointment nurse on the phone. And you feel pressed to tell the doctor how many boxes of Kleenex or bottles of cough medicine you've been through to prove that despite this mirage of good health, you really are sick.

One could argue that in the natural course of the infection, you coincidentally began to get better the same day you went to see your doctor. After all, your body had a week or more to subdue this pest. But it's likely that the mere act of calling to make an appointment with a doctor—a ritual your mind and your body probably associate with getting better—helped you heal. Instead of feeling chagrined and foolish that you can no longer muster dramatic evidence of your illness, you should be feeling proud that you and your body are powerful enough to produce the medicinal results of a doctor's visit without even seeing the doctor.

This is one of the most commonly experienced examples of the placebo effect, which I hope to rename remembered wellness. My first serious look at remembered wellness came in 1975, and I'll admit that the reason I delved into the phenomenon was to answer critics who suggested that the relaxation response I had defined was "nothing but the placebo effect." I was sure that the relaxation response was a distinct physiologic state that had to be brought forth by specific means and not "willed" into being by belief. So in truth it was my disdain for the placebo effect, and the fact that some had lumped my findings with what were considered arbitrary emotional reactions, that motivated my initial investigations.

I found that there was little research on the phenomenon. Researchers had generally ignored it, rarely making mention of

it in articles in medical journals. Most considered the phenomenon an irritating variable, a fluke that didn't merit scientific study. Nevertheless, the existing research was impressive.
Much of the evidence of the power of remembered wellness
had existed for decades but had not been promoted in the
medical community. Most investigators relied on the 30 percent
success rate that Dr. Henry K. Beecher of Massachusetts General
Hospital attributed to the placebo effect in his 1955 study. Even
though there were indications that the placebo effect was far
more powerful, only a handful of researchers had returned
for a closer look. We'll take that closer look ourselves in this
chapter and the next.

It was on the basis of the evidence presented here that I began asking why remembered wellness occurs and what mechanisms make it work. I began to question my assumptions and
the medical community's assumptions. I learned that the
placebo effect worked much better than we usually appreciate,
and that there were three routes to activating human beliefs.

Subjective Versus Objective

Before I get to the data, let me take a minute to discuss
subjective and objective results of remembered wellness.
I will emphasize the existence of significant objective
findings in this book because remembered wellness will never
be accepted into standard medical practice and into Western
society without "measurable results." Three requirements
must be fulfilled before a scientist can establish an objective,
scientific result: measurability, predictability, and reproducibility. These are the standards that medical science uses
to gauge the merits of any research study and that the National Institutes of Health Office of Alternative Medicine has
recently begun to apply to unconventional treatments to separate proverbial snake oil from proven, helpful therapies.

The effects of remembered wellness are measurable, but because remembered wellness is activated by the individual's
unique set of beliefs, its effects are not easily predicted or re-

produced. We can look at groups of people who have benefited from placebo therapy and offer overall rates of success. But at this time, our tests and measures are not sensitive or sophisticated enough to gauge the individual preferences and life experiences that are at play in each incident of remembered wellness.

Of course, as we will see in the examples of this chapter and throughout the book, medicine is almost never purely objective, because both caregivers and patients possess biases and beliefs. Some would argue that mind/body medicine will prove science's inadequacy to answer all the questions about human life that we expect it to. But we don't have to throw the baby out with the bathwater. I think that science will eventually be sophisticated enough to predict and reproduce some belief-engendered effects. What we call "personal" will be considered powerful, and researchers will pursue commonalities among diverse people rather than the unrealistic quest for universality we employ today. Then, the individualistic nature of this influential healer—remembered wellness—will change the way we practice medicine.

Researchers *can* achieve objective assessments by using unbiased technology and mathematical formulas. In my career I have been continually amazed to see that beliefs do generate these kinds of quantifiable results. Nevertheless, I don't want to denigrate the subjective—what people think and feel—in emphasizing the value of objective measurements. Beliefs manifest themselves differently in the body, and while some beliefs bring about results the profession can measure in test tubes, blood pressure cuffs, or with electronic monitors, others produce symptoms that are real in their effect on patients but perhaps cannot be tracked by our current technologies.

Traditionally, doctors have thought that if a symptom could not be measured, it must be fake or nonexistent. We've distrusted a patient's ability to perceive authentic bodily change. But my research and that of many others has demonstrated that perceptions and physicality are very tightly braided together in the body, so it is impossible to separate objective and subjective change.

Granted, it is easier to attend to and respect symptoms that we can measure and monitor. But as our understanding of the brain grows, we now realize how much *more* there is to measure and track, and how pale our technologies look when compared to this intricate, ever-changing organ, the human brain. Even though science cannot now measure most of the myriads of interactions entertained in the brain, we should not ignore compelling brain research that demonstrates that beliefs manifest themselves throughout our bodies. I'll present the evidence of this in an upcoming chapter. But for now, let me introduce you to the research studies that catapulted my explorations of remembered wellness.

Better Than We Knew

I n 1979, my colleague Dr. David P. McCallie Jr. and I reviewed a long history of therapies designed to alleviate angina pectoris, pain in the chest and arms caused by decreased blood flow to the muscle of the heart. The treatments, ranging from injections of cobra venom to surgeries to remove the thyroid or parts of the pancreas, were enthusiastically introduced into medical practice years ago even though today we know they were misguided. But despite there being no physiologic reason these techniques should have worked, they often did. When these ersatz techniques were used and believed in, they were effective 70 to 90 percent of the time, working two or three times more often than Dr. Beecher had said they would. And interestingly, later, when physicians began to doubt whether these treatments worked, their effectiveness dropped to 30 to 40 percent.

Nevertheless, our 1979 findings fell on deaf ears. My colleagues greeted the subject with skeptical interest but remained wedded to the more routine approach to illness, preferring to rely solely on medications and procedures. Then, more recently, the placebo effect began to attract more attention. In 1994, Dr. Alan H. Roberts and his colleagues of the Scripps Clinic and Research Foundation looked at medical and surgical treatments of bronchial asthma, herpes simplex cold sores, and duodenal ulcers. Employing a retrospective approach, as

Dr. McCallie and I had in studying angina patients, Roberts's team studied treatments once thought to be successful but later debunked. They concluded, according to *Clinical Psychology Review,* that "under conditions of heightened expectations" the power of the placebo effect "far exceeds that commonly reported in literature." A full 70 percent of the patients they studied experienced excellent or good results from bogus treatments.

In a subsequent study, chief investigator Dr. Judith A. Turner of the University of Washington, Seattle, also confirmed that the placebo effect was twice as effective as commonly thought. Dr. Turner's team evaluated the role of remembered wellness in relieving pain, reviewing three books and seventy-five articles published over fifteen years. Calling the success rates "strikingly high on average," Turner said clinicians must no longer assume that placebos work only one-third of the time.

So the first step in establishing remembered wellness was to at least double our expectations of how well it worked. Physicians could no longer dismiss the phenomenon as a relatively minor factor, because now it seemed to have an effect the *majority* of the time. Remembered wellness was found to have a substantial impact on the most commonly reported symptoms—chest pain, fatigue, dizziness, headache, back and abdominal pain, numbness, impotence, weight loss, cough, and constipation. And, as demonstrated in a 1992 Ohio State University study of patients with congestive heart failure, placebo treatment may also help more serious conditions. In that investigation, patients with moderately severe cases who received eight weeks of placebo therapy proved capable of an eighty-one-second improvement in their mean duration on an exercise treadmill.

Three Components
of Remembered Wellness

I t is easy to harvest the benefits of remembered wellness. Over twenty years ago, Dr. Mark D. Epstein and I identified three different but often overlapping ways to achieve the

---

TABLE 1

THREE COMPONENTS OF REMEMBERED WELLNESS

1. Belief and expectancy on the part of the patient
2. Belief and expectancy on the part of the caregiver
3. Belief and expectancies generated by a relationship between the patient and the caregiver

---

phenomenon, all of them dependent upon beliefs. Belief in or expectation of a good outcome can have formidable restorative power, whether the positive expectations are on the part of the patient, the doctor or caregiver, or both (see Table 1).

To see how the patients' beliefs trigger remembered well-ness, take a look at Dr. Stewart Wolf's 1950 study of women who endured persistent nausea and vomiting during preg-nancy. These patients swallowed small, balloon-tipped tubes that, once positioned in their stomachs, allowed researchers to record the contractions associated with waves of nausea and vomiting. Then the women were given a drug they were told would cure the problem. In fact, they were given the op-posite—syrup of ipecac—a substance that causes vomiting.

Remarkably, the patients' nausea and vomiting ceased en-tirely and their stomach contractions, as measured through the balloons, returned to normal. Because they *believed* they received antinausea medicine, the women reversed the proven action of a powerful drug. Even though many of us stock our medicine cabinets and first aid kits with ipecac to bring about vomiting in case of poisoning, these pregnant women with documented stomach distress thwarted the ac-tion of a drug that should have made them even sicker. With beliefs alone, they cured themselves.

Similarly, a 1957 investigation at Cook County Hospital in Chicago found that 30 percent of patients with rheumatoid arthritis benefited from placebos. Their relief persisted at least three months. This was confirmed and enhanced by a 1995 study published in the *Annals of Internal Medicine* in which 40 percent of patients with rheumatoid arthritis experienced at least a 50 percent decrease in the number of swollen joints and a 50 percent reduction in swelling and tenderness that existed in joints. Simply relying on placebos, they found their improvements lasted six months or more.

Another investigation centered on people who had their lower wisdom teeth removed. For three to four decades, dentists have used ultrasound frequencies transmitted through a small, hand-held device called a transducer to massage a patient's face after surgery to reduce pain and swelling and to hasten healing. But dentistry does not know of any physiologic reasons why this technique works. In 1988, a team of dental surgeons in London compared the experiences of postoperative patients who received no ultrasound treatment to those receiving ultrasound massages as well as to those who got mock treatments in which the ultrasound machine was kept at zero frequency. For one mock treatment, the doctor held the transducer motionless on the patient's face, while in the other treatment the doctor moved the transducer in circles on the patient's cheek. Yet another set of patients was asked to massage their own cheeks with a disconnected ultrasound transducer. Prior to surgery, all the groups of patients were assured that the use of the ultrasound would reduce postoperative pain and swelling.

When the results were tabulated, patients who received the mock nonmassaging treatment had 35 percent less swelling than did those who received no treatment at all. Patients treated with the mock circular treatment and the actual ultrasound massage had 30 percent less swelling compared to the control group, but those performing self-massage with the disconnected transducer had only a 15 percent reduction.

If you've had wisdom teeth removed, you'll undoubtedly recall wanting to wish away the proverbial chipmunk cheeks. But in this case, the patients' desires did have results; they believed in the prospect of a helpful technology, which mobilized their internal healing resources.

Having a clinician administer the treatment also seemed to make a difference in the healing process, since patients who performed self-massage had less success. In the research my colleague and I did on angina pectoris, we also found that the contribution of the caregiver's beliefs was impressive. Indeed there was a direct correlation between the enthusiasm conveyed by the physician investigator and the success rates. As long as a therapy was professed to be the latest and the greatest, the vast majority of patients experienced excellent effects. Eventually, when the treatments were shown to be ineffective, they fell out of favor and improvements in patient health correspondingly declined.

Not only did patients report subjective relief from their pain, they displayed objective improvement—greater endurance in exercise tests, less use of nitroglycerin, and improved results on the electrocardiogram. Some of the patients enjoyed this objectively documented improved health—mind you, this was after receiving what would later be declared a worthless treatment—for a year or more.

If we take a more conservative approach and only consider those angina patients who had coronary artery disease confirmed by a diagnostic angiogram, 60 to 80 percent of the study participants achieved substantial relief of symptoms. Applying the wisdom of the Framingham Heart Study in which only 14 percent of men and 19 percent of women experienced spontaneous remission after suffering angina for two or more years, spontaneous remission cannot begin to account for this success rate.

Clearly, when patients *believed* in therapies that were fervently recommended by their doctors, this fervor worked to alleviate a variety of medical conditions including angina, asthma, herpes simplex cold sores, and duodenal ulcers. But as soon as patient confidence in these treatments was undermined, so was the effect. This is the pattern noted by the nineteenth-century French physician Armand Trousseau when he said, "You should treat as many patients as possible with the new drugs while they still have the power to heal."

The Pleasing Placebo

Learned in childhood, the act of pleasing others often has its own rewards, including health benefits, as is suggested by the word "placebo," from a Latin root meaning "I shall be pleasing or acceptable." Most health professionals and patients are eager to please one another, the former by being friendly, hopeful, and confident in the therapies being recommended, and the latter by getting better, by reporting improvements in health, or by complying with instructions.

Throughout history, society has afforded healers a special deference and admiration. We undoubtedly do this because we so ardently need for them to work magic and produce miracles. But in modern times, we've removed the aura we used to associate with healing. We've come to expect only facts and figures from our doctors, not hocus-pocus, and lately we don't even count on their succor and reassurance, as did previous generations. We disapprove of the deference people paid to physicians years ago, and we try to eliminate the intimidation factor many patients feel when they talk to their doctors. But in the process we may have depreciated our expectations of healers—the same expectations Hippocrates, the father of Western medicine, knew were important to our healing when he said, "Some patients, though conscious that their condition is perilous, recover their health simply through their contentment with the goodness of the physician."

Too often today, the sacred trust that should be developed between doctor and patient has been replaced by a set of rushed interactions. The therapeutic rewards a good relationship engenders are lost in an age when patients are discouraged from visiting their doctors. Researchers conducted an investigation at Massachusetts General Hospital in 1964 that warned us all about the importance of this bond. They compared two matched groups of patients who were to undergo similar operations. The doctor responsible for their anesthesia visited both groups of patients but interacted with them quite differently. He made only cursory remarks to patients in one group but treated the other group with warm and sympathetic attention, sitting on the patients' beds, detailing the steps of the operation, and telling them about the pain they might expect afterward.

The patients went on to have their operations and to recover. They were allowed to have as much pain relief medication as they requested. The hospital personnel caring for them either did not know to which group the patients belonged or were unaware that the test was being conducted.

The relationship established by the anesthesiologist made a tremendous impact. The patients who received the friendlier, more supportive visits got better faster and were discharged from the hospital an average of 2.7 days before patients in the other group. (This was, by the way, in the days before insurers determined the length of hospital stays.) And the patients treated in a warm and sympathetic manner experienced less pain, asking for half as much pain-alleviating medicine as the other group.

I digress for a moment to offer a personal example of the influence a caregiver can have on a patient's health. A young woman, whose internist consistently measured high blood pressure readings when she was at his office, had consistently normal-range readings when she visited me. She marveled at the difference, saying, "Dr. Benson, I'm never nervous when I visit you." I was, of course, flattered until further questioning revealed the true source of her occasional hypertension. When I asked her why she got flustered in her other doctor's presence, the patient replied, "He's so cute!"

This is but one example of "white-coat hypertension," a medically recognized phenomenon in which fear—or in my patient's case, infatuation—temporarily elevates blood pressure in the doctor's office. Indeed, physicians and caregivers can have a profound effect on us. British researcher Dr. K. B. Thomas posed the question "Is there any point to being positive?" in his 1987 study published in the *British Medical Journal*. His research team examined the effects of the doctor's conveyance of positive or negative information to two hundred patients with symptoms not attributable to any particular physical ailment. These patients accounted for 40 to 60 percent of the visits to the clinic the researchers studied. In the positive consultations, the doctor gave patients firm diagnoses and confidently remarked that they could expect improvement in a few days. Sometimes, patients received prescriptions that the doctor told them would make them better when in fact the prescriptions were really vitamins. In other cases, no prescription was given and the doctor told patients none was required.

In the negative sessions, the physician stated, "I cannot be certain what is the matter with you." Offering no medication, the doctor said, "Therefore I will give you no treatment." When the doctor supplied a prescription, again in the form of vitamins, he or she told the patient, "I am not sure that the treatment I am going to give you will have an effect." The appointments closed with the doctor telling a patient to return to the clinic if he or she experienced no improvement in the next few days.

In the end, 64 percent of the patients who heard good news got better within two weeks of the consultation compared to only 39 percent of those who received negative feedback. The weight of a doctor's words was proven all the more consequential because statistically there was little or no difference between those who received prescriptions and those who didn't. About 53 percent of patients given vitamins got better in the two-week span compared to 50 percent of those who received none.

The Manner Matters

The bedside manner does matter. I have often heard patients say, particularly when referring to surgeons or other specialists, that proficiency is more important to them than bedside manner. But in examples cited here from both medical and surgical wards, it's plain that a positive, supportive approach is an essential part of the healer's proficiency. No matter how precise the surgery, studies show you'll recover more quickly if your surgeon is upbeat, confident, and kind.

The patient too has responsibilities in cultivating a good re-

lationship with the health professional. Audiotaping patients'
visits with their doctors, Drs. Sherrie Kaplan and Sheldon
Greenfield at New England Medical Center in Boston determined that the average patient asks fewer than four questions
in a fifteen-minute meeting with the doctor, and those queries
include, "Will you validate my parking?"

Trying to improve communication, the researchers coached
patients with chronic illnesses such as diabetes, rheumatoid
arthritis, and high blood pressure prior to their regularly scheduled doctor appointments. The coaches spent twenty minutes
with patients, going over their medical records and focusing on
questions the patients wanted to ask once they were with their
doctors.

Not surprisingly, the coached patients came away from
their visits better satisfied than the uncoached group. But in a
more dramatic development, coached patients experienced
fewer illness-related limitations to their lifestyles than did uncoached patients. Patients with diabetes who more actively
conversed with their doctors had lower follow-up glucose levels, a sign of better diabetes control.

In every incident of remembered wellness, the catalyst is
belief. The belief may be your own, a composite of your life
experiences. The belief may be your clinician's, the product
of his or her professional and personal history. Finally, the belief can be instilled in you by the confident and trusting tone
established in consultations between the two of you. As humans we are laden with beliefs, influences so interwoven we
cannot precisely distinguish their sources. Spurred by a remote childhood memory of a congenial pediatrician who re-
warded you and your brother with a toy after every checkup,
you may be predisposed to expect rewards from medicine. Or
conversely, if you remember hating needles so much as a child
that it took your mother, several nurses, and the doctor to
hold you still for a shot of penicillin, your prejudices may be
long-standing.

The Nocebo Effect

Y ou see, belief can also work against us. The brain/body does digest unpleasant images and can fulfill ugly prophecies. Consider how often crime victims die from heart attacks, brought on not by any injuries but from the horror of being assaulted. Confirming this, one investigator autopsied such victims and observed that in eleven of fifteen cases there were no internal injuries. Instead, their deaths were caused by severe heart muscle damage called myofibrillar degeneration. Jolted by believing in a life-threatening danger, the body sustained this damage, releasing excessive amounts of the stress-relieving hormone norepinephrine, also called noradrenaline. A massive overdose of norepinephrine triggers a chain of biochemical events, often causing death.

The nocebo is the placebo's negative counterpart, and just as our bodies can remember wellness, they can also project sickness and even death. Western medicine tries to account for the materialization of beliefs into physical signs and symptoms by calling such illnesses "psychosomatic."

The formation of "psychosomatic medicine" departments in the 1940s was meant to foster a better understanding of how, for example, episodes of anger and hostility can translate into stomach ulcers and heart attacks, but because medicine separated and compartmentalized the realms of mind and body for so long, the discipline never got the respect it deserved. In the long run, this may have been for the best since no one discipline can address the vast interrelatedness of mind and body. Every specialty and subspecialty of medicine is having to reevaluate and appreciate how intimately our thoughts are related to our bodies. Even songs are going to have to be rewritten, since it isn't just a matter of the thigh bone being connected to the hip bone, it's a matter of our everyday thoughts, dreams, and superstitions being related to our entire anatomy.

Voodoo

No example better illustrates the relationship between mind and body, or the paralyzing power of negative beliefs, than does voodoo death. Voodoo is a set of religious practices believed to have originated in Africa that is still being practiced by native populations in Africa, Haiti, South America, and the West Indies. Some aboriginal tribes in Australia, New Zealand, and the Pacific Islands have a similar set of beliefs and practices.

Many voodoo deaths have been documented in the medical literature. Witch doctors in Australian aboriginal tribes are known to "point a bone" to cast a spell on an intended victim. This rite is supposed to so disturb the spirit of the victim that disease and death will result. In 1925 Dr. Herbert Basedow witnessed such an incident and wrote:

> The man who discovers that he is being boned is, indeed, a pitiable sight. He stands aghast, with his eyes staring at the treacherous pointer, and with his hands lifted as though to ward off the lethal medium, which he imagines is pouring into his body. His cheeks blanch and his eyes become glassy, and the expression of his face becomes horribly distorted. . . . He attempts to shriek but usually the sound chokes in his throat, and all that one might see is a froth at his mouth. His body begins to tremble and the muscles twist involuntarily. He sways backwards and falls to the ground, and after a short time appears to be in a swoon; but soon after he writhes as if in mortal agony, and covering his face with his hands, begins to moan. . . . His death is only a matter of comparatively short time.

Dr. Walter B. Cannon, the famous Harvard Medical School physiologist at the turn of the century, found tremendous power in "tapu," or taboo, in the Maori aborigines of New Zealand. When tapu was wielded against others by the tribal chiefs, Cannon said it produced "a fatal power of the imagination working through unmitigated terror."

Cannon recalled one story in which a young aborigine stayed at an older friend's home while traveling. For breakfast, the elder served a meal containing wild hen, a food that the younger generations were strictly prohibited from eating. The young man asked his host several times if his breakfast contained wild hen but was assured it did not.

A few years later, these friends were reunited, and the older man asked the younger if he would now eat wild hen. The young man said that of course he would not because it was forbidden. The elder laughed at him and explained that years before he had tricked him into eating the hen—news that caused the younger man tremendous fright and eventually physical distress. Within twenty-four hours, he was dead.

In the late 1700s, Dr. Erich Menninger von Lerchenthal of Vienna reported several instances of sudden death brought on by extreme fright. One of the cases he cited came from Joseph Haydn's diary in which the composer wrote:

> On the 26th of March at the concert of Mr. Bartholemon (London) there was an English clergyman who while hearing my Andante sank into the deepest melancholy because of the fact that on the previous night he had dreamed of such an Andante which announced his death. He immediately left [our] company, went to bed, and today I heard through Mr. Bartholemon that this clergyman had died.

The same doctor reported a gruesome tale of an assistant who was widely disliked by students at a college. The students condemned the assistant to a mock death ceremony in which the man was restrained and held down while his head was placed on a chopping block and his eyes were blindfolded. One student simulated the sound of a swinging ax while another dropped a wet, warm cloth on the assistant's neck. The shock was so great that the assistant died immediately.

Similarly, Dr. George Engel, recently a professor of psychia-

try at the University of Rochester Medical Center, found that
extreme feelings of hopelessness and helplessness, or what he
termed the "giving up–given up complex," produced sudden
death. We see frequent examples of this in widows and widow-
ers who get sick right after the deaths of their spouses, and we
say that these people "die from a broken heart."

Dr. Engel found one hundred examples of sudden deaths in
unusual circumstances in newspaper clippings from around
the world, and by re-creating the psychological status of those
people before their deaths, he found that an individual's sense
of powerlessness and an inability to cope with life often led to
that person's death. Engel concluded it isn't the circumstances
of life but one's attitude toward these circumstances that seals
one's fate.

A forty-five-year-old professional man exhibited this characteristic hopelessness before his abrupt demise, according to
Dr. Leon J. Saul of Media, Pennsylvania. The man was evidently
torn between staying in an intolerable situation at home or
moving to a new town and leaving behind responsibilities he
felt he should shoulder. Haunted by the demons apparent to
him in either choice—to stay or go—he boarded a train to
make the move to the other town. But about halfway between
his old home and his new home, the train made a stop where
the passenger disembarked and began pacing along the platform. When the conductor called "All aboard!" the man could
not decide what to do and in fact was convinced he could travel
no farther. At the height of this emotional impasse, he collapsed on the train station platform and died. His medical
records indicated no significant or life-threatening illness.

The faith or faithlessness that governs our lives can affect
our health. The nocebo effect occurs in the same three ways
as does remembered wellness, whenever beliefs, faith, or expectations are at play. Correspondingly, the use of placebos in
experimental studies not only produces positive effects, it can
also generate unwanted side effects, some of which can be severe. Drowsiness, headaches, nervousness and insomnia, nausea and constipation are among the most commonly reported
side effects of placebo treatment, according to Dr. Raymond

C. Pogge, who conducted a review of seventy-seven publications for the incidence of placebo side effects.

About 33 percent of placebo recipients in a test of antispasmodic drugs experienced nausea or constipation. When participants received placebos in a trial of pain-relieving medications and tranquilizers, 8.9 percent of them felt drowsy as a result. Six patients had documented cases of liver impairment after taking placebos. In one study a patient got a skin reaction from a placebo; the reaction disappeared upon discontinuance of the placebo and reappeared when it was administered again.

Reading the informed consent document one has to sign before participating in a double-blind study is undoubtedly the culprit in some of these cases. Knowing a long list of potential undesirable and toxic effects may bring them on. Similarly, if you associate previous bad experiences with certain medications, or know that the drug being tested should make you tired or sick to your stomach, you may trigger these very symptoms even if you are ingesting a sugar pill.

Pseudopregnancy

In remembered wellness and the nocebo effect, the adage "Be careful what you wish for" is profound. Women, and in rare cases men, who either desired or feared pregnancy intensely, or empathized keenly with someone who was pregnant, have been known to show actual signs of pregnancy. This phenomenon is called pseudocyesis and is often considered "the oldest known psychosomatic condition." Hippocrates reported twelve cases of women "who imagine they are pregnant seeing that the menses are suppressed and the matrices swollen." In the sixteenth century, Mary Tudor, the Queen of England, experienced pseudocyesis several times with symptoms of pregnancy that spanned nine months and culminated in two episodes of false labor.

These pseudopregnancies have also been documented in modern times. In a 1951 study by Dr. Paul H. Fried and his colleagues at Jefferson Medical College and Hospital in Philadelphia, the symptoms were so convincing that a fifth of the doctors declared a third of the patients "pregnant." In this condition, menstruation stops and abdominal swelling occurs at a rate similar to that of a normal pregnancy. Breasts grow larger and more tender, and nipples change pigment as is consistent with pregnancy. Nipples also increase in size and milk is secreted. Some women feel what they think is fetal movement during the fourth or fifth month of a false pregnancy. Dr. James A. Knight of Baylor University reported that one man had a false pregnancy as well.

Many patients who had false pregnancies were found to be depressed as a result of a failed romance or infertility. Depression then had unmistakable effects on the brain and thus on the pituitary gland and hypothalamus. With the mental focus on pregnancy mimicking that of a pregnant woman, the brain was persuaded to process orders for hormonal changes in the body even when no developing fetus was present.

Longing for a baby. Longing for an absent loved one. Longing for renewed health and vigor. The body does respond to the cravings of the soul, sometimes in dramatic ways, other times subtly. The body even responds to what our caregivers want for us and to the trust we build in relationships with our caregivers. Faith, that is, longing and expecting that what we long for will occur, helps our bodies recall the messages and instructions associated with what we long for. In other words, a doubting Thomas may stunt remembered wellness. Take the case of two thousand men who were treated with beta-blocking drugs after having heart attacks. It turned out that doubts or negative beliefs, translated into actions, helped determine whether they lived or died.

Following Doctors' Orders

Reported in a 1990 paper in the British medical journal *The Lancet*, the investigation compared the effects of beta-blockers, drugs that prevent hormones from causing the heart to beat too rapidly or forcefully, to the effects of placebos. The study revealed that men who did *not* adhere well to the treatment regimen—whether they received active medication or inert placebos—were 2.6 times more likely to die within a year of follow-up than were good adherers. It didn't matter whether these men were taking the beta-blockers or placebos; if they took the pills less than 75 percent of the time, they were *twice* as likely to die as those who took the medicines or sugar pills more consistently. Remarkably, the death rate among those who did not take their placebos was much higher than for those who took their placebos regularly!

A similar result was revealed in an investigation of men who received either a cholesterol-lowering drug or placebo after having a heart attack. This study, published in *The New England Journal of Medicine*, revealed that after five years of follow-up, only 15 percent of those who took 80 percent or more of their placebos died over that time compared to 28 percent of poor adherers taking placebos. Again, not taking a placebo led to an increased rate of death.

As medical researchers, we expect some exceptions and anomalies from our statistics. But the finding that patients who consistently followed doctors' orders, believing that doing so would make them well, were twice as likely to live is sobering. The sacred trust appears all the more sacred, the responsibility for fostering positive outlooks and a willingness to adhere to treatment all the more consequential.

Now you've seen some of the objective medical evidence that first compelled me to take remembered wellness seriously. Reading these studies and conducting my own, I learned that our systems are nourished or starved according to our expectations. When mobilized for our benefit, this is a magnificent physiologic endowment. And in the next chapter we will see that it is the nature of belief to affect the natural course of our lives.

CHAPTER 3

THE NATURE OF BELIEF

Having examined the research results you've just read, I began to see the prevalence of remembered wellness, a common thread that weaves its influence into our minds, bodies, and into healing itself. But to call it a physiologic truth, I had to know: "Are all of us equally susceptible to remembered wellness and the nocebo effect?," "Which beliefs are important?," and "How might health-influencing beliefs be formed?" These are the questions I'll address in this chapter as we develop a deeper understanding of the beliefs and preferences we all, very naturally, entertain in life.

Does It Work for Everyone?

Researchers have tried to determine whether or not it takes a certain personality, sex, age, or level of intelligence to experience remembered wellness or the nocebo effect. We'll talk more about these factors throughout the book, but in general these studies contradict one another or fall short of definitive answers. I believe this is because we are all capable of remembered wellness or the nocebo effect, since we are all wired to exhibit beliefs in physical ways. Timing and stimuli appropriate to the patient may heighten the effects of remembered wellness, in the same ways timing and certain stimuli heighten the effects of medications or other therapies. And the initial dose of a drug or placebo often produces a more significant effect on patients than subsequent doses.

Seventy-four percent of the complaints patients bring to medical clinics are of unknown origin and are probably caused by "psychosocial" factors, according to a study reported by Dr. Kurt Kroenke of the Uniformed Services University of Health Sciences in Bethesda, Maryland, and A. David Mangelsdorff, Ph.D., MPH, of the Brooke Army Medical Center in Houston, Texas. Other studies indicate that between 60 and 90 percent of all our population's visits to doctors' offices are stress-related and probably cannot be detected, much less treated effectively, with the medications and procedures on which the medical profession relies almost exclusively. In other words, the vast majority of the time, patients bring medical concerns to the attention of a healing profession that cannot heal them with external tools or devices. Instead, doctors must rely on patients' internal mechanisms. Much of the success the medical profession achieves is not due to anything doctors do or dispense that is inherently healing. We should really attribute the success of many medical treatments to the inherent healing power within individuals.

But this isn't how physicians typically handle these situations. Co-editor of *Mental Medicine Update,* Dr. David S. Sobel, MPH, reports in the newsletter the story of a woman who goes to see a third doctor after many months of suffering from numbness and weakness that was severe one day and nonexistent the next. The symptoms were not confined to one area, traveling to different body parts. The first two doctors had told her, "It's all in your head," at worst making the condition sound like a figment of her imagination and at best suggesting that she was not effectively managing the stresses of everyday life.

The new doctor did a complete workup and extensive testing at the end of which she was told she had multiple sclerosis, an incurable disease that can slowly destroy the nervous system, eventually causing death. But when the doctor told her this diagnosis, she responded, "Oh, I'm so relieved, I thought it was all in my head."

This is a very unsettling story. The woman appears to have been very poorly served by our profession. Western medicine still makes serious distinctions between mental, emotional, and physical roots of illness despite the amassing of research that finds that mind and body are so interwoven that such distinctions are not only artificial, they're unscientific. Strikingly, having symptoms deemed psychological is such a humiliating experience in our society that the woman preferred to have a debilitating and life-threatening disease.

Doctors tend not to sympathize with beliefs and imaginings that may be stirring the body to action in ways an outside observer cannot measure. Instead of helping patients to mobilize beliefs to produce healing, physicians either reassure people—an act that can be soothing if a patient believes the assurances—or dismisses them, leaving patients feeling either frustrated or embarrassed for complaining in the first place. This frustration or embarrassment may, in fact, encourage patients to "prove" their illness to doctors—a desire that their bodies could eventually fulfill in more demonstrable health problems.

When doctors diagnose an illness as being "in your head," they seem to be saying that you imagined the problem, and that it is not real or authentic. Far greater credence is given to the molecular menagerie inside of people and to diseases that have technical, impressive names, not to mention the tangible evidence on which health professionals rely to make informed decisions. Even psychosomatic medicine, the study of disease that is brought on by beliefs, limited itself to the tangible or measurable, the signs doctors and nurses could point to and say, "Yes, illness is actually occurring."

It's no coincidence then that droves of patients are turning to unconventional healers who, often by definition, have a greater respect that not all illness can be seen or documented. (Of course, it is the very lack of evidence that makes their practices questionable and the potential for abuse and fraud so enormous.) Indeed it is estimated that Americans spend $13.7 billion annually on unconventional therapies, presumably to meet a need traditional medicine does not adequately address or fulfill. But as cognizant as traditional medicine is of the public's increased reliance on unconventional therapies, the system will not change dramatically without proof that these therapies are truly good for patients. As scientists, we must distinguish the inherently healing qualities of these treatments from the success of the treatments made possible by remembered wellness. But to a certain extent, by focusing on the inherent healing qualities or risks of homeopathy, aromatherapy, or herbal treatments, medicine is missing the more important point—that beliefs can be a major source of illness and a major force in treatment.

This point will only be brought home to medicine with scientific evidence like that which we reviewed in the last chapter. In those cases, patients who suffered from diseases ranging from herpes simplex cold sores to duodenal ulcers to angina pectoris were found to be able to help themselves because they expected—but did not actually receive—valid pharmacological or technological assistance. As we saw in pregnant women who reversed the action of ipecac and in the documented tragedies of voodoo death, the power of belief is mammoth. With medicine beginning to acknowledge untapped sources of healing— beliefs that produce objective results—perhaps greater attention will be given to the unseen, yet undetected, consequences of belief, those that comprise the majority of complaints patients bring to doctors. Nevertheless, all of us entertain beliefs that make a difference in our physical health.

Obvious Influence

Although our medical training does not encourage us to do so, physicians do instinctively know—and if they practice medicine for any length of time, observe— ways in which their patients' beliefs and expectations shape outcomes. For example, it has long been common knowledge that participants in drug trials or research studies get better faster and have better results than other patients. The socalled Hawthorne effect, named for the factory where the phenomenon was identified, occurs in patients in research studies, in participants who are receiving active medications or treatments, as well as in those receiving placebos. Researchers attribute the Hawthorne effect to the fact that caregivers pay more attention to patients participating in studies and more enthusiastically anticipate the results.

Remembered wellness makes its presence known in many facets of patient care and in many departments within hospitals. One need look no further than the surgical ward to see that doctors instinctively understand—and sometimes allow their decisions to be influenced—by the power of certain intangibles, the patient's fears and imaginings, for example. Most surgeons prefer not to operate on patients who are convinced they are going to die during surgery.

My friend Dr. Thomas P. Hackett, since deceased but once the chairman of the Department of Psychiatry at Massachusetts General Hospital, and his colleague Dr. Avery D. Weisman published a paper in 1961 that revealed the results of three years of studying patients who were about to have surgery. By interviewing patients beforehand, they found that six hundred were unusually apprehensive about the procedure while only five of those patients were convinced that their deaths would occur while on the operating table. Correspondingly, most of those termed unusually apprehensive survived while none of the latter did.

In each of the five cases in which patients had a predilection to death, Drs. Hackett and Weisman wrote, "Death held more appeal for these patients than life because it promised either reunion with lost love, resolution of long conflict, or respite from anguish." Obviously, these patients were so affected by the burdens of their lives that they predicted death and their bodies delivered it.

Few experiences in life stir as much anxiety in people as major surgery. But in the same way that mind/body interactions work against us, self-care techniques can work for us. The Reverend Dr. Edmond Babinsky, director of pastoral care at the Medical Center of Central Massachusetts, tells me that he taught Ann Burgess, a thirty-five-year-old admitting clerk in his hospital, to meditate to quell her anxiety before surgery for a blood clot in her leg. Ms. Burgess had had a very bad experience with anesthesia in a previous surgery and she told Dr. Babinsky that she "just couldn't face the idea of the operation."

Knowing that she was Catholic, Dr. Babinsky introduced the subject of eliciting the relaxation response and gave her a laminated card on which the steps for eliciting the response were printed. He also gave her a "meditation stone," a white pebble Dr. Babinsky picked up from a beach on Cape Cod. (He often brings back pebbles for his patients.)

Ann Burgess went through the surgery with flying colors, and she attributed part of the success to the phrase she said to herself as she was wheeled down the hallway from her hospital room to the operating suite. "Be still my soul," she said, again

and again, her fingers wrapped around the stone her friend
the chaplain had given her.

Expectations and Preferences Intervene

You see, a patient's positive frame of mind can be ex-
ceedingly therapeutic. In 1986, Drs. Carole Butler and An-
drew Steptoe at the University of London used two
competing powers of suggestion in their study of asthmatics. The
asthmatics' breathing ability deteriorated significantly after in-
haling what they believed to be a chest-constricting chemical. But
if the patients had been treated beforehand with what they believed to be a powerful new bronchodilating or chest-expanding
drug, they had no such deterioration. In both instances, the patients received inert, distilled water. Thus, bronchial constriction
was caused by belief and prevented by belief.

From Western Australia comes an investigation that demonstrated that patients who have spinal tap diagnostic procedures
get headaches when they are warned beforehand that
headaches may occur. Although the physiologic reason for
them is unclear, headaches have long been an expected side effect of the test, in which a syringe inserted between the verte-
brae of the back is used to take cerebrospinal fluid. But in
1981 in Kiribati, formerly the Gilbert Islands, at a time when the
spinal tap was relatively new to the practice of medicine in that
region, investigators found that when patients were not warned
that headaches might occur, only one in thirteen reported this
side effect within twenty-four hours of having the procedure.
Seven of fifteen patients told to expect headaches afterward reported having headaches over the same time span.

But influential beliefs can be introduced to us in many different ways, and not necessarily in medical settings. Who
would imagine that something as seemingly irrelevant as one's
favorite colors could affect medicine? A mode of interior design that is becoming popular around the world, feng shui is a
system of colors and symbols that the Chinese believe evokes
certain reactions and vibrations within us. Fans of feng shui

maintain that the careful selection of colors and placement of furnishings will, for example, enhance the success of a business establishment by connecting with and fulfilling the customer's unconscious preferences and reactions. Some people also use the design principles in their homes.

Indeed, color does seem to affect the way we perceive and absorb the benefits of medicine, although definitive studies must still be pursued. Investigators from the University of Alabama found that white pills are usually associated with analgesic or pain-relieving action, lavender with hallucinogenic effects, orange and yellow with stimulant or antidepressant action. On the other hand, some colors did not seem to imply particular effects: dark green was found to be a weak choice for implying pain relief, black weak in implying stimulant, and blue did not imply depressant or sedative. Italian researchers found that patients with sleep problems benefited more from blue capsules than orange capsules and that to a certain extent preference depended on the sex of the patient. A British rheumatologist found that red was the most effective color for pain relief in treating rheumatoid arthritis.

Form also seems to affect function, according to a University of Alabama study that revealed that patients believe capsules are more powerful than tablets. A 1972 *Lancet* study also showed that in placebo treatment two capsules produced more changes than one. In another study, patients responded better to sweet-tasting placebos than to bitter-tasting ones. We don't yet understand the full logic behind the preconscious biases our brain attaches to our sensory perceptions. But our influential expectations and ideals are also formed in response to the people, environments, and challenges we encounter in life. Culture and ethnicity inspire many tenets of our lives. So, fascinatingly, our upbringing may determine how much pain we experience.

Cultural Differences

It's long been known that individuals vary in their ability to withstand pain. But several studies demonstrate that beliefs formed in our socialization contribute to our threshold for pain. In 1965, Dr. Richard A. Sternbach and my mentor, Bernard Tursky of Harvard Medical School, summarized the findings of previous investigations of attitudes toward pain among "Old Americans" (defined as Protestants of British descent), Jews, Italians, and the Irish:

> Each group has its own configuration of attitudes towards painful stimuli and towards the expression of responses to pain. . . . Old Americans have a phlegmatic, matter-of-fact, doctor-helping orientation; Jews express a concern for the implications of pain, and they distrust palliatives; Italians express a desire for pain relief; and the Irish inhibit expression of suffering and concern for the implications of the pain.

Dr. Sternbach and Tursky conducted their own study in which sixty women, then termed "housewives," of Old American, Irish, Jewish, and Italian descent received electric shocks to their forearms to test their perceptions of and ability to withstand pain. Old Americans were defined as those with parents and grandparents who were born in the United States. The Irish, Jewish, and Italians were those whose parents had been immigrants to the United States.

Consistent with previous findings, the investigation revealed that Italians tolerated pain the least and focused more on the immediacy of the pain. Jewish participants, on the other hand, were almost as sensitive to pain but were more likely to be concerned with the future implications of pain, the way the shocks might affect them later despite assurances that no permanent harm would occur. Old Americans adapted to pain more readily, verbalizing for doctors an attitude of needing to "take things in stride." The Irish, who had similar endurance and adaptability to pain, described "keep[ing] a tight upper lip" at the same time as they "feared the worst."

In chronic or long-term pain, such as that associated with arthritis or lower back strain, a 1993 study reaffirmed the findings that ethnicity affects perception and thus the intensity of pain. And Dr. Maryann S. Bates and her colleagues later documented that Hispanic patients reported the highest intensities of pain, followed by Italians. In contrast, Polish and French Canadians had the lowest pain scores, with Old Americans and Irish in the middle. (Asian, African, and Native Americans were among ethnic groups not addressed in these particular studies.)

None of these investigations was meant to create or reinforce stereotypes. Rather, the scientific evidence is meant to show us that pain is only pain as we know it. Our upbringing and our heritage contribute to our perceptions of pain and, thus, our ability to endure it. The importance of these studies lies in the relationship not just between socialization and perception of pain but between perception of pain and the reality of pain. Your perceptions, the collection of impressions "in your head," are the reality. Because perceptions have real outcomes, your pain cannot be singularly attributed to an arthritic joint or a strain in your lower back. Instead the full constellation of influences, including the traditions of your ethnic group and culture, must be taken into account.

My mother had a medical experience that illustrates this point beautifully. Raised in the Orthodox Jewish faith, Mom is in her mid-nineties, although because she so often fibs about it, her age is a matter of ongoing dispute. She is a very active woman, walking miles every day and following up her jaunts with yoga exercises in the apartment she maintains, still living on her own. But fifteen years ago, Mom began to have fainting spells, the result of a narrowing of her heart valve, which sometimes happens with age. At the time the fainting spells ensued, Mom was still an active golfer and more than once had to be retrieved from the links by ambulance.

Despite my being a physician—or perhaps tacitly because I am—Mom avoids all medical evaluation and eschews taking medications except at the insistence of family. But once she was diagnosed, Mom was sternly advised that she needed an aortic valve replacement, an operation that would ensure the free flow of blood from her heart into the aorta and thence to her entire body. My mother reluctantly agreed to the surgery in which a valve from a pig's heart was to replace her damaged valve. The surgeons also took veins from her leg to conduct four coronary bypasses of clogged arteries.

After this very complex surgery, doctors found that she was bleeding internally. So within a day of the first surgery, Mom was operated on a second time. In all, she required twenty-two units of blood.

She awakened after these ordeals two days later, lying amidst a web of draining pumps and tubes, intravenous lines, and connections to heart monitors and oxygen catheters located on either side of her bed. I asked Mom how she was feeling, and she replied with an irritated and insistent "I'm nauseous." I tried to reassure her: "Of course you're feeling nauseous. You've been through two major operations." My mother looked me in the eye and waved me quiet. Then she indignantly pointed to her chest and uttered one important word—"Pig."

Having never consciously consumed pork in her ninety-some years, Mom reported ill effects not from the trauma of surgery but from the idea that she had profoundly violated a religious mandate. I sought the hospital's rabbi to assure her this was not a violation, and he told me that it was not uncommon for Jewish patients to feel uneasy about the pig valve procedure. When my mother received his blessing that the operation represented no lapse in her observation of religious traditions, her nausea quickly subsided. Today her heart remains healthy and she is back to her regular routine, outwalking everyone her age.

Taboos Made Manifest

From the time we are babies, our parents, our teachers and school friends, our churches, our governments, and our communities feed us information about what to fear and avoid, and about actions that would be detrimental and/or undesirable. We don't realize that these lessons are physically translated. We are taught to look both ways before crossing streets and to stay away from configurations of three shiny, pointed green leaves with red stems. Just as we are warned about poison ivy, Japanese children learn to stay far from lacquer and wax trees because of potential allergic reactions. And Japanese investigators Drs. Yujiro Ikemi and Shunji Nakagawa were fascinated by the fact that patients who merely walked under lacquer or wax trees, or by factories that process lacquer, developed severe rashes and other symptoms of dermatitis including burning, itching, and swelling.

Skeptical that minute amounts of the wax or lacquer could cause such reactions, Drs. Ikemi and Nakagawa launched a study in which fifty-seven high school boys were tested for their sensitivity to the allergic substances. The boys filled out questionnaires about any past experiences with or sensitivities to the poison trees, other allergies, and their families' allergy histories. The boys were then divided into groups based on the severity of reaction they claimed to have had in the questionnaires.

Boys who reported marked reactions to lacquer trees in the past were blindfolded and on one arm were brushed with leaves from a lacquer tree that they were told were leaves from a chestnut tree. They were brushed with chestnut tree leaves on the other arm but told the leaves were from the lacquer tree. Within minutes, the arm the boys believed to have been brushed with the poisonous tree began to react, growing red and developing bumps, causing itching and burning sensations, while in most cases the arm that had actual contact with the poison did not react.

The researchers concluded that the reaction of patients depends on constitutional factors, such as the susceptibility of the skin to a toxin and the amount of the toxin, and the effects of suggestion, or what a patient thinks about the toxin. But in 51 percent of cases, suggestion was a more powerful force than were the constitutional factors. Skin reactions indistinguishable from actual allergic reactions were induced by *believing* contact with a poison had occurred.

Beliefs About Pain and Disability

Increasingly I've come to reject long-held notions of biology being separate from belief. Neither can be completely isolated to demonstrate its prowess; these forces are indivisible. Look at a 1988 study conducted at Brown University by Dr. John F. Riley and his colleagues. They determined that patients diagnosed with symptoms of chronic pain were more likely to be impaired, despite the severity of pain they reported, if they believed that pain implied impairment.

Dr. Riley's team observed that patients with chronic pain often exhibit a disability that "pervade[s] all aspects of their lives" and are often "unable to engage in gainful employment." Patients with chronic pain often find themselves experiencing chemical dependence, emotional distress, marital and family disruption, and vocational difficulties, and it is common for them to overuse the health care system in their repeated and often frustrating attempts to gain relief from their pain.

The investigators surveyed fifty-six patients who experienced pain in various parts of their bodies—the mean duration of their pain was 35.1 months—on their attitudes toward pain and disability. They asked the patients to keep diaries of their pain, and they tested the patients' physical strength and mobility. In the end, independent of the pain levels reported, those who believed pain should inhibit their movement were the most inhibited. In other words, the belief that pain implies disability has more to do with disability than the pain itself.

The team argued that the health care profession may contribute to the downward cycle experienced by chronic pain patients by introducing and reinforcing the belief that being pain-free is the ultimate goal. In truth, chronic pain is rarely cured completely. Dr. Riley and his colleagues summarized that health care workers may teach patients "to attribute impairment to pain, whether directly (e.g., with instructions to take it easy when in pain) or indirectly (by treating pain complaints with acute pain relief interventions)." Medicine—and a society that is bombarded with advertising offers of quick fixes and miracle cures—may be cultivating impairment by promoting an undue expectancy of pain relief. Instead, emphasis should be placed on increasing activity and mobility.

When fed images of disability and despair, the body is wired to accept these limits as truthful and to respond with impairment. This is the nocebo effect. If instead the body absorbs images of activity and mobility, as if it sees flashcards in a word association game, the body literally reconfigures its vision of itself. This is remembered wellness.

Every moment your brain is introduced to reams and reams of new information and beliefs, a dynamic and ever-constant stream of inputs from both inside and outside the body. These inputs are not just sights and sounds, temperatures and smells, food and oxygen, but prayers and original thoughts, books you read or talks you have over coffee with friends, reassurances from your doctor or directives from your boss, the touch of a lover, or the cheer of a crowd at a football game. The extraordinarily complex brain and its cohorts within the nervous system not only assess the inputs but change, literally reconstitute themselves, as a result of recording or "remembering" these internal and external inputs. And every instant, this process goes on and on and on.

Perceptions Become Reality

However, our brains often cannot distinguish external from internal "reality." When you dream that you are being chased, your heart rate increases just as it would if you were really being chased. For your brain, and thus your heart, this is reality.

I remember seeing the movie *Lawrence of Arabia* in a movie theater in 1962. Because the film was lengthy, it was shown in two sections with an intermission in between. I'll never forget the crowd's crazed convergence on the concession stand and the immense demand for beverages during the intermission after what had been nearly two hours of exposure to hot, dry, desert scenery. I later found out that record numbers of beverages had been sold during that movie. Of course we're all accustomed to getting choked up in sad movies, or having rushes of adrenaline, also called epinephrine, and increased heart rates in violent or suspenseful films, but it was impressive to see actual, demonstrable thirst, no different from what would have been true had all of us actually been in the desert alongside Peter O'Toole and Omar Sharif.

Beliefs can bring on severe reactions. I'd hazard a guess that all of us have heard stories about people dying on or around their birthdays or other personally significant occasions. In medicine, this phenomenon has become known as the "anniversary reaction." Plato and Buddha are said to have died on their birthdays. Forefathers Thomas Jefferson and John Adams both died on the fiftieth anniversary of the signing of the Declaration of Independence. Known to have been a rival of Jefferson, John Adams spoke the final words, "Thomas Jefferson still surv—?" Jefferson's last words were, "This is the Fourth?" Till their last breaths, and perhaps ensuring their last breaths, Jefferson and Adams held on to beliefs that shaped their entire careers and lives, not to mention the birth of a nation.

In their aptly titled paper, "The Birthday: Lifeline or Deadline?," Dr. David Phillips and peers at the University of California, San Diego, reported that a study of over 2 million people revealed that women are more likely to die in the week following their birthday than in any other week of the year. In contrast, deaths among men peak just before their birthday, suggesting that the birthday is a kind of deadline for males. Women, the authors argue, are more likely to believe that birthdays are joyous celebrations in which relationships with people they care about are renewed. Men, on the other hand, may view birthdays as times to take stock of their accomplishments, as deadlines by which they were to have achieved certain goals. With their beliefs, women appear able to prolong life to enjoy these occasions, while men may succumb out of dread of the upcoming deadline, or out of a desire to beat the deadline.

Famous people appear to be able to circumvent both these effects. Dr. Phillips's team believes this is because they are more likely to receive positive attention on their birthdays and because they feel more confident about their accomplishments.

Other investigations have demonstrated that deaths among Chinese people fall before the Chinese new year and rise immediately afterward, as happens with Jewish people before and after Passover. Another study shows that a woman may experience great psychological and physical distress on reaching what would have been the due date of an aborted fetus.

Traumatic Events and the Nocebo Effect

Difficult and traumatic events carry with them fantastic power. *The New York Times* featured a story of a woman who went deaf after the Kobe, Japan, earthquake of 1995. Although no physiologic reason for deafness was available, the woman lost her hearing after enduring the screams of help from a neighbor, a veterinarian trapped in a building's rubble. The woman had yelled to the man in the rubble that she would help him escape but left to help others first because the veterinarian assured her he was all right and could wait. But before she could return to him, a fire broke out and engulfed the veterinarian's building. The woman could do nothing but stand by helplessly as the man's shouts escalated in desperation and eventually subsided in agony. Her only mode of coping was to will herself deaf.

Our brains are wired for beliefs and expectancies. When activated, the body can respond as it would if the belief were a reality, producing deafness or thirst, health or illness. Antonia Baquero, the patient I talked about in the first chapter who was so adversely affected by the removal of calcium deposits from her breast, went on to have a belief suggested to her by an untrustworthy source. And although she'd made great progress in remembering the calm and confidence that she had maintained before the surgery, another person's opinion of her caused a setback.

A while after she began eliciting the relaxation response and enjoying the serenity of her mother's Spanish prayer, Ms. Baquero left the country to live in Hong Kong for several months. While she was there, friends encouraged her to come along with them to see a Chinese medical practitioner. Upon first seeing her, the practitioner told her that he read her face and that she did not look well. She remembers, "He told me to take certain herbs. I was very upset. Here I was in a foreign country, away from my doctors. I panicked and again felt that I was losing control." Her anxiety at the prospect of cancer returned.

Feeling tremendous distress, Ms. Baquero called me from

Hong Kong. She recalls that I told her not to give credence to this out-of-the-blue medical assessment. As she remembers, "Dr. Benson told me to put the herbs in the toilet or to throw them away. He was emphatic. And I trusted him. As uncomfortable as I was, I trusted the way he had said it. A year later, I went back to see the Hong Kong practitioner who had frightened me, and he told me he had been quite ill and that he had been careless in his diagnosis. When I thought about how adamant he had been, I realized I could really have been damaged." The observation that Ms. Baquero did not look well played upon her worst fears, prompting a fleeting recurrence of the anxious symptoms that had bothered her months before. Her belief in another opinion restored her well-being.

Ms. Baquero chose to have more faith in health than in illness. Today at age forty-six, she reports that she is in excellent health, running three to four miles three times a week, enjoying yoga classes, and taking no medicines. She no longer panics over the risk of cancer.

It's a physician's responsibility to encourage good nutrition and exercise, to discourage smoking and its devastating effects, to oversee medications, and to advise patients on healthy lifestyle decisions. This includes encouraging an appetite for positive, hopeful expectations and steering patients away from beliefs that can be destructive, and from those who would take advantage of and manipulate a patient's beliefs, putting their own gain before the patient's welfare.

Again, this is a role most physicians and other health care practitioners instinctively understand and sometimes even value. I'm sure it was this same kind of instinct that caused my discomfort with the repercussions of diagnoses. We've seen that an individual's beliefs can markedly affect their health and that a physician's reassurance can make a measurable, physiologic difference. Now we'll examine the brain mechanisms that transmit remembered wellness and permit beliefs to make such an impressive mark on our health and well-being.

CHAPTER 4

THE BRAIN'S PREROGATIVE

The psychologist and philosopher William James once said that "if there is anything [that] human history demonstrates, it is the extreme slowness with which the academic and critical mind acknowledges facts to exist [that] present themselves as wild facts, with no stall or pigeonhole, or as facts [that] threaten to break up the accepted system." Dr. James couldn't have been more apt in describing Western medicine's slow digestion of mind/body research.

Stalls and pigeonholes have inhibited our progress. And in my attempt to remain as objective and detached as the accepted system requires, I did what some people think is a strange thing. Even though, together with collaborators, I published scientific articles establishing the safety and efficacy of the relaxation response more than twenty years ago, I refused to elicit it myself on a regular basis until just five years ago. Now it would be silly for a scientist to prove the health benefits of a new and harmless drug but refuse to use it for himself when needed. But the value of self-care and remembered wellness are much harder sells to the scientific community, and I had to be sure that I kept enough distance from my research to maintain credibility with my colleagues and patients.

To prove to others that mind/body interactions were real, and that medicine should be taking advantage of these connections to heal people, I needed to remain objective. I believed that this kind of conservatism was warranted because medicine typically considers studies of the body important and groundbreaking, while research into people's minds and beliefs is deemed unworkable or inconsequential.

This dichotomy between mind and matter can be traced to thinkers as far back in history as Plato. However, these differences were best articulated by the seventeenth-century French philosopher and mathematician René Descartes. Descartes was the first to suggest that the body did not need the mind to function, heightening respect for the machinelike qualities of the body that have become the dominant focus of contemporary Western medicine.

But the lenses of modern technology have finally enabled us to report on the similarities and interrelatedness of mind and body. I've summarized relevant, new information about the brain in this chapter. With these clues, I began building on my hypotheses that all human bodies foster an internal healing power.

Dr. Antonio R. Damasio is a pioneering brain researcher from the University of Iowa. In his superbly written and scientifically profound book *Descartes' Error*, Dr. Damasio chides Descartes for retarding the biological understanding of the mind—an effort he says has really just begun—and for inspiring the peculiar way in which Western medicine studies and treats disease. He suggests that if Western medicine is to improve, it can no longer exclude from consideration the physical roots and repercussions of mental functions. He writes:

> This is Descartes' error: the abysmal separation between body and mind, between sizable, dimensioned, mechanically operated, infinitely divisible body stuff, on the one hand, and the unsizable, undimensioned, un-pushpullable, nondivisible, mind stuff; the suggestion that reasoning, and moral judgment, and the suffering that comes from physical pain or emotional upheaval might exist separately from the body. Specifically: the separation of the most refined operations of the mind from the structure and operation of a biological organism.

The Decade of the Brain

Almost as if to compensate for past irreverence, former President George Bush by U.S. presidential proclamation declared the 1990s "the decade of the brain." And brain science has never been so prolific. But even in light of all we have learned, the brain—on average a three-pound glob composed of about a quart of gelatinlike tissue—remains largely mysterious. In appearance, it is split down the middle into two distinct spheres, and to a certain degree, although less than neurologists originally thought, mental and physical functions can be traced to local areas of the left or right side of the brain.

The brain is so complex, so constantly in motion, so mega-faceted and super-connected that all our attempts to describe its actions are, by nature, simplistic. Every remarkable discovery we make only further elucidates how astonishingly powerful and elaborate is the brain and its circuitry—that which affords us life and health, movement and memory, intuition and wisdom. The brain is, after all, comprised of approximately 100 billion neurons or nerve cells (see Figure 2). At a

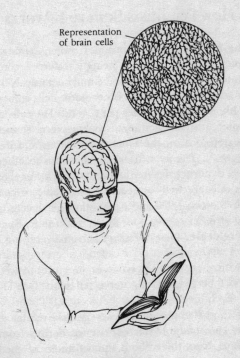

Representation
of brain cells

FIGURE 2
THE BRAIN MAGNIFIED

Peering into a magnification of the substance of the brain, you'd see a multitude of nerve cells. There are, in fact, over 100 billion nerve cells in your brain.

microscopic level, these nerve cells are communicators, expressing messages to and fro. But bundled together in groups—and these groups congregating in even larger groups—nerve cells form a macrocosm, a brain divided into regions that have identifiable controls and functions, one ensuring our sight while another registers emotions, one allowing us to flex our muscles while others regulate the beating of our heart. The faculties we usually think of as "the mind," interpreting signals and deciding what they mean to us, emerge from this macrocosm.

How Scientists Believe It Works

The brain is an extraordinary switchboard with immense numbers of calls being transferred, connected, interpreted, and returned simultaneously. Nerve cells "fire" or transmit messages to other nerve cells constantly, at rates of hundreds of messages per second. The cells come in microscopic, three-dimensional puzzle-piece shapes, with stringy extensions on the ends called axons and dendrites (see Figure 3). The axon transmits messages to other nerve cells while dendrites receive the inputs from other axons.

Nerve cells are well-connected beings, able to communicate with between 1,000 and 6,000 other nerve cells, making about 100 trillion connections at any given time. But the axons do not deliver these messages personally, relying instead on a kind of chemical courier called a neurotransmitter. Axons emit these chemicals at synapses, junctures between dendrites and their neighboring nerve cell axons (see Figures 3 and 4). Each nerve cell has between 1,000 and 500,000 synapses. Every thought you have, every move you make, every sensation and emotion you experience derives from these connections, from the trillions upon trillions of encounters between axons, neurotransmitters, and dendrites that occur every fraction of a second, every hour of the day as brain messages are formulated, sent, and received.

More than fifty different neurotransmitters have so far been

identified. In this book we have already referred to the neurotransmitter adrenaline, which acts, in part, to stimulate the
heart's beating as happens in the fight-or-flight response. Some
neurotransmitters are linked to disorders—as dopamine is with
schizophrenia and serotonin with mood swings—but nevertheless neurotransmitters are crucial players in normal brain
function, transferring messages to and from the myriad of
nerve cells.

To further complicate matters, each synapse can communicate at different strengths, the same way a voice can communi-

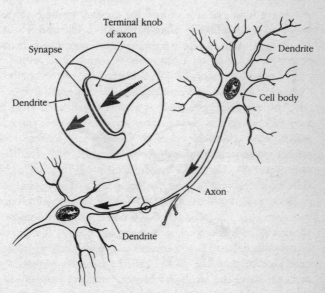

FIGURE 3
NERVE CELL COMMUNICATION

*Isolating a few of the billions of the brain's nerve cells in this diagram, you'll
see that they feature cell bodies, dendrites, and axons. To communicate between
the cells, axons transmit messages from the cell body. These messages cross a
juncture, the synapse, and are carried to the dendrites of other cells. The insert
is a representation of one synapse. The arrows indicate the direction of the message being transmitted. Every millisecond of your life, trillions upon trillions of
these messages are sent and delivered by this extraordinary system in your brain.*

cate at different volumes. Professor Paul M. Churchland of the University of California, San Diego, writes in his book *The Engine of Reason, The Seat of the Soul*, "If we assume, conservatively, that each synaptic connection might have any one of 10 different strengths, the total number of distinct possible configurations of synaptic weights that the brain might assume is, very roughly, 10 raised to the trillionth power or $10^{1,000,000,000,000}$."

When You Burn Your Finger

Here is an example of how the message-routing system works. Suppose you are lighting a candle and let the match burn too low, burning your finger. The pain-at-

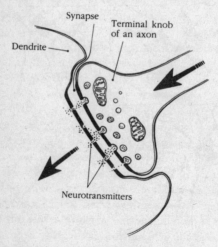

FIGURE 4
SYNAPSE CLOSE-UP

The small specks being released at the synapse represent neurotransmitters, the messenger chemicals that travel from the axon of one cell across a synapse to be incorporated into a dendrite of another nerve cell. Depending on the amount of neurotransmitter released and the receptivity of the dendrite responding to the neurotransmitter, different gradations of messages are capable of being transmitted.

tuned nerve cells in your finger react, axon upon axon sending signal upon signal, all via neurotransmitters crossing a multitude of synapses to express the message from your finger to your spinal cord to the mindful regions of your brain. These distinct regions of the brain, not all of them yet identified or understood, are responsible for certain actions—one interprets pain messages and orders pain relief to the rescue, another gauges the emotional importance of the event and triggers emotional reactions.

But no matter how the nerve cells mingle, no matter what synapses are crossed, no matter what regions are targeted, the brain retains a memory of the nerve cell activations and interactions associated with the event of burning yourself. With every event, billions upon billions of these events being processed by the brain at any given time, nerve cells conspire to provoke a plethora of responses. All of this happens in tiny fractions of seconds!

The brain responds to and interprets messages from three different sources: the environment, the body, and the brain itself. So, when you burned yourself, your brain registered what burned you—the match—as well as what the body experienced—injury—and what the mind experienced—pain and unpleasantness. Forever recorded in your brain is an image of the incident—a representation of the environmental factors that contributed to the problem, the physical impact, the emotional impact, and the particular circuitry of nerve cells that handled the multitudinous messages evoked by the incident.

Our senses are obviously responsible for recording many of the details of an incident that go into the files our memories maintain. But the sense that is particularly keen and dominant in one person may be much less active in another. As you probably already know, some of us are very visually oriented, so that, for example, seeing the froth of an incoming wave on a beach, or seeing the words on this page, registers more distinct impressions in the brain than would be true of an auditory-oriented person, who needs the sound of the wave surging in or a tape of these words to make the most profound impact in his or her mind.

I try to accommodate these different sensory tendencies in my treatments. For example, to elicit the relaxation response, I teach patients to focus on something that pleases them. It doesn't matter if it is a tape of forest sounds, a postcard of a beach they went to last summer, a piece of paper on which an inspirational phrase is printed, the smell of an incense they recall from church, or the feel of their sneakers padding the pavement as they jog. They will cull the greatest impact, and probably adhere to the practice of mental focusing because they enjoy it more, if they "focus" in ways that feel natural to them and their brains.

The act of focusing your mind on a visual image is called a "visualization." I often recommend that people recall some very soothing, beautiful place they have been to, maybe on a vacation, or maybe someplace comforting they remember from childhood. Similarly, I recommend that people use "affirmations," positive messages that people repeat either out loud or quietly to themselves, after they have finished eliciting the relaxation response. In both of these instances, the idea is to introduce a new sensory idea into your brain, especially when your brain is accustomed to a stream of negative thoughts or self-criticisms.

Our sensory leanings may also explain some of the reasons people are drawn to New Age symbols and unconventional therapies, and why some people find aromatherapy particularly soothing while others buy crystals. As we'll continue to see, when you know how to plug into them, the wirings of our brains can be very influential.

No matter how you stimulate the brain, the details of the experiences you have, and all the senses you use, are registered in your brain. That which appears to be a crude clump of jelly assembles and then retains notes on every movement, every breath, every incident that has ever occurred to you or ever will, as well as every thought and dream you have ever had or ever will have. And as we will discuss in greater detail, it also carries the wisdom of the ages—guidelines gained over an evolution of human life that promote your survival.

Bottom-Up, Top-Down

Burning a finger is "a bottom-up" event, as is the viewing of a pretty landscape (see Figure 5). Science has long appreciated that the brain was capable of interpreting "bottom-up events"—of responding to stimuli from the environment or from the body itself. Only recently has brain research revealed that "top-down" events are also possible. Top-down events originate in your thoughts (see Figure 6). They are either memories of events that your brain recorded before, or new thoughts you bring to mind. Imagine that you take a burning match in hand weeks after the initial accident, or that you remember the beautiful landscape months after you

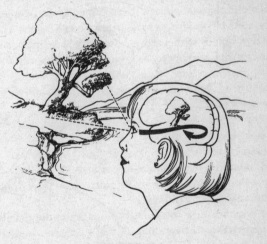

FIGURE 5
A BOTTOM-UP EVENT

The woman observes a pastoral scene. The scene is external to her body, but through the action of her nerve cells becomes a registered image and then a stored memory in her brain. Since the scene started outside of her brain, not from the "top," that is, in her thoughts or imagination, it is called a "bottom-up" event. Other bottom-up events originate in our bodies—in sensations in our fingers, stomachs, ears, or noses.

first saw it. In the case of the match, your memory of burning
yourself could be vivid enough to trigger a thought-induced
flashback and a projection of the distress you originally felt.
And similarly, remembering the landscape, you'll experience
the same wash of peacefulness you originally felt upon viewing
it. The brain tends to interpret these top-down messages the
same way, as if the imagined or projected scenes were real.

Top-down events are common. Have you ever been driving a
car and imagined an accident occurring? You probably emerge
from this momentary lapse only to realize that your speed has
decreased and that your heart rate has increased. Without the
environmental stimulus of an actual accident, of screeching

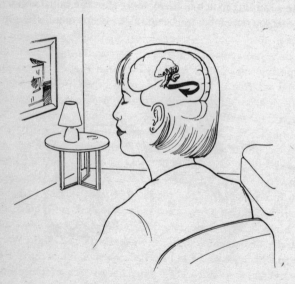

FIGURE 6
A TOP-DOWN EVENT

*The woman is sitting indoors with her eyes closed, imagining the same pas-
toral scene she viewed previously. Her brain reconstructs the image stored in
her memory by re-creating the pattern of nerve cell activity that occurred when
she actually viewed the scene. But now this image originates from inside her
brain, from her thoughts and memories. This is a "top-down" event. Dreams
are also top-down events.*

tires or cars slamming against one another, without the physical impact of such an event, your nerve cells have nevertheless reacted. Your mind has ordered the same fight-or-flight response it would have for the real threat of an accident, and unbeknownst to you has directed your foot to ease off the gas pedal.

Vivid Memories As Triggers

I n the same fashion, memories can trigger very powerful top-down events. When I was an intern in Seattle, at what was then the King County Hospital, I had a powerful experience with the fight-or-flight response, a reaction so strong that it looms large in my memory. One day I was working in a walk-in clinic in which people with common, nonemergency medical problems were evaluated. An Asian man in his sixties came into my office, and I had an overwhelming, instantaneous reaction to him. I broke into a sweat, I felt nauseated, and my heart started beating rapidly. I experienced unmitigated fear of this man for no reason I could identify.

I quickly regained my composure, took a medical history, and examined him. At the end of the examination, I confessed to this patient, "I don't believe I know you, but I had this very intense and strange reaction upon seeing you when you first walked into the room." The man smiled, extended his right hand in a fist, pressing his thumb up and down, and in a menacingly familiar voice, declared, "Okay, Yank, now you die!" He explained that in the early days of World War II he was the actor who had played the part of Tokyo Joe in Hollywood pictures, which I told him I had seen as an impressionable six- or seven-year-old. The scene he reenacted in the examining room was one in which he played a fighter pilot who, with his plane's machine gun, shot down American planes and their pilots. He always played villains, he told me, and went on to be cast in Charlie Chan movies, scores of which I also saw as a kid.

Stored in my subconscious, deeply buried where I could not unearth them, were memories so potent that his appearance in my clinic activated my fight-or-flight response. This man posed no threat to me, but my body reacted as if this villain had strode right off the movie screen into the walk-in clinic in which I worked, the danger palpable and immediate.

Movie Magic

Movies will come up now and again in this book, and I suspect that is because I am a visually oriented person on whom movies make a tremendous mental impact. We're used to thinking of movies as powerful because they're played on big screens, in dark theaters, with audiences that react en masse. But I encourage you to begin to think of movies, television, and all the external ticklers in your life in a profoundly different way. When you consider how the brain works, and you understand that the information you feed it changes your biological structure and affects your health and well-being, as I will continue to demonstrate in this chapter, your life's stimuli will seem much more important. It often takes the realization of a physical impact for Western society to understand the importance of intellectual and spiritual stimuli.

I know that, in my case and in the cases of many others, moving pictures are so vivid that we feel like we know actors and actresses because their images and scripts become physically materialized in our brains. They literally become a part of who we are. And as you'll see in a moment, when we talk about the incredible influence of emotion on the processing and prioritizing of thoughts, depending on the emotions these actors inspire in us, they become players in a cognitive world in which we project images of ourselves that change the physical signals traveling through and instructing our bodies.

Virtual reality is another powerful stimulus. These video games and tools are often being used in ways that seem to blur the lines between bottom-up and top-down thought processes. For example, physicians now help patients get over acrophobia, a severe fear of heights, using virtual reality helmets so patients can view, explore, and step to the edges of computer-generated bridges, buildings, and diving boards—the height of which appears to be quite dramatic. I don't mean to make a pun by applying bottom-up and top-down terminology here, but with the aid of virtual reality, these patients can record bottom-up events in their brains—near height experiences, if you will. Gradually, as a result of these near height experiences, the top-down event, or thought, of having to go to the fortieth floor of a building, may not provoke as much anxiety. Nor will future experiences with actual heights be so traumatic. I understand that after virtual reality treatment, one patient took a hot-air balloon ride, soaring above the earth and enjoying every minute of it without fear or physical distress.

My collaborator Marg Stark and her husband had their first experience with virtual reality at a local amusement park when they conquered a slalom run that had been filmed on an actual Olympic race course. They were strapped into seats in a dark booth that lurched and swayed right along with the film that was projected, always threatening to hurl them into a crowd of spectators or over a cliff. Although the booth's jerks and sways were not raucous enough to hurt them, both Marg and her husband experienced muscle fatigue in their backs and legs—similar to that which they have had after a day of skiing. And they were ravenous afterward, their metabolism seemingly spurred into action by the virtually real physical challenge they had endured. Their bodies were mobilized because their brains could not distinguish real physical challenges from computer-generated ones.

The Act of Remembering Wellness

The scenes we recall or imagine are, indeed, real to the brain. Dr. Stephen M. Kosslyn, a colleague of mine who is a professor of psychology at Harvard, conducted an experiment in which persons were asked to look at a grid, a box of interconnecting parallel and horizontal lines. While they did so, Dr. Kosslyn and his fellow researchers used a type of X-ray called a PET scan (positron-emission tomography), one of the new lenses of technology I referred to earlier, to determine the areas of the brain in which the nerve cell activation occurred. PET makes it possible to view the brain in action because patients receive a very small dose of radioactive substance that zeros in on the increased blood flow indicative of increased nerve cell firing. With the help of these scans, Dr. Kosslyn's team identified the hotbeds of brain activity brought about when participants gazed at a grid.

Then the picture of the grid was taken away and the participants were asked to close their eyes and envision the grid from memory. As they did, another set of PET scans were taken. The second scans revealed that the same areas of the brain were put to use, the same hotbed of cell firing instigated by seeing a grid was brought on by remembering but not actually seeing the grid.

Thus, an image is formed when a certain constellation of nerve cells are activated. To recall an image, the brain reconstructs the constellation of activity that first occurred. Patterns of brain activation are stored and remembered: To revive a memory, in this case a remembered visual grid, the brain calls on the same actors—nerve cells, synapses, and circuits—that converged originally to view the grid. This pattern of brain activity needed to recall such an image is sometimes called a "neurosignature." All of our life events and emotions have neurosignatures, shorthand notations the brain stores and recalls. With notation upon notation about system upon system, our brains and nervous systems entertain a constant dialogue that cultivates and maintains our life memories, emotions, personalities, even our ethics and morals. And because all of our lives are different, each of us has unique, unequivocally unique, neurosignatures.

The Incredible Power of Emotion

We are unaccustomed to thinking of emotions and personality traits being biological in nature. We think emotions come to us and over us quite arbitrarily. We think personalities form over the course of life experiences, not because certain circuits in the brain get used a lot, locking us into particular patterns of brain activity and behavior. But this is what the latest brain research is revealing. Emotions are the natural outgrowths and representations of the brain as it takes into account a full picture of the body and the world around it. And they are far more important in brain function and in deciding our health than our society, which promotes objective reasoning, ever knew.

How would emotions figure into the rapid-fire communiqués sent between body and brain that occurred in the example in which you burned a finger? Most of the time you will be able to go on and light candles and fireplaces and barbecue grills in the future without being inhibited by fear. The fact that you can do that despite the environmental stimulus of the presence of fire and the memory your brain retains of the impact of the previous burn is, in part, because your emotions help your brain weigh the importance of these events, persuading the brain that this is an unremarkable event for which there is no need to mobilize its resources in preparation for a burn.

To start with, scientists believe that some emotional reactions enter into brain activity *before*, not after, we've had some time to think something over and decide what we feel about it. Psychologists have developed a test to assess these instantaneous reactions. They introduce people to pictures, sounds, and words, about which people declare immediate likes or dislikes. They also introduce nonsense words, such as "juvalamu," which has proved intensely pleasing to people, and "chakaka," which was despised by English speakers.

"We have yet to find something the mind regards with complete impartiality, without at least a mild judgment of liking or disliking," reports Dr. Jonathan Bargh, a New York University psychologist who has studied the way the brain entertains emotions, in a recent article in *The New York Times*. Dr. Bargh contends, "People evaluate everything as they perceive it," assigning emotional values even to things they've never encountered before such as abstract shapes and nonsense words.

"This is all part of preconscious processing, the mind's perception and organization of information that goes on before it reaches awareness," Dr. Bargh explains. And because these judgments happen in a fraction of a second and become a part of our first impression, he says, "we trust them in the same way we trust our senses," unaware that we have already adopted a bias. Thus, he and other scientists conclude that there is no such thing as objectivity, only objective thinking that arises from a subjective mind.

Synesthesia

Emotion has also been implicated in the neurologic phenomenon synesthesia, which Washington, D.C., neurologist Dr. Richard E. Cytowic describes in his book *The Man Who Tasted Shapes: A Bizarre Medical Mystery Offers Revolutionary Insights into Emotions, Reasoning and Consciousness*. Only ten of every one million people on earth are synesthetes, who, because of their conscious awareness of a normal brain process, are apt to say that a piece of chicken tastes round, that a symphony sounds green, or that a chime is chocolatey.

When they do so, synesthetes seem to consciously tap into what is an unconscious, physiologic process for most of us or the preconscious processing I have described—the bringing together and sorting out of signals or impressions—that our brains entertain dynamically all of the time. In other words, at the first bite of chicken, or even at the first whiff of it cooking, a synesthete may recognize the cognitive shuffle going on in the brain, the senses that are sorting themselves out and being ordered around.

Dr. Cytowic says that emotion acts like a valve, deciding what will grab our attention and what will not. But emotion has a "logic of its own," so we may not be able to predict how our brains will "tag" perceptions. Guided by what Dr. Cytowic suspects are their unique emotional impulses, synesthetes—whom Dr. Cytowic calls "cognitive fossils"—are compelled to consciously process multisensory events, which most of us have lost the ability to do. And most importantly, because of these brain properties, he suggests that self-awareness is only "the tip of the iceberg" of who we really are. "What we think of as voluntary behavior, set in motion by free will, is really instigated by another part of ourself." Thus he concludes:

> We know more than we think we know. The multisensory, synesthetic view of reality is only one thing that we are sure has been lost from consciousness. There could be a lot more. If you want to try to reclaim some of this deeper knowledge, I suggest that you start with emotion, which to me seems to reside at the interface between that part of self [that] is accessible to awareness and that part which is not.

In this book, we will talk a great deal about this inner knowledge, about intuitions and emotions and how to respect them in a society that encourages you not to. But for now, it's enough to settle on the fact that emotions are not whims of an intangible soul. They are instead dispatches of the brain as it interprets the body's experiences in everyday life, both the challenges of the physical environment and the values, concerns, and stories that enrich our encounters. They play a far more crucial role in our physiology than most of us realize.

Some of the most important clues to the contribution emotions make in the brain have been gained by neurologists who observed the dispassionate way in which people with prefrontal lobe injuries (just behind the forehead and above the eyes) approach life after sustaining damage to their brains. A patient Dr. Damasio refers to as Elliot in long passages in *Descartes' Error* had an orange-sized tumor removed from his brain and forever after approached life with tremendous detachment. Prior to the surgery, he was a good husband and father with a steady job in business; after the surgery, he could not keep a job, he invested in risky business ventures and went bankrupt, divorced his wife and married another woman, a relationship that quickly ended in divorce. Trying to get at the cause of this upheaval, Dr. Damasio had Elliot undergo a battery of tests. In one test, Elliot looked at and responded to photos of emotionally charged subjects such as houses burning or people drowning in floods. Although Elliot knew the images would have disturbed him prior to his surgery, he felt little or no emotion about them in his postsurgical state.

About this incredible transformation, Dr. Damasio writes, "the cold-bloodedness of Elliot's reasoning prevented him from assigning different values to different options, and made his decision-making landscape hopelessly flat." Intrigued by the fact that both Elliot's ability to feel emotions and to make reasonable decisions were impaired, Dr. Damasio began to focus on the brain's mechanisms of rational thought, discovering that emotions contribute to one's decision-making by assigning values to certain memories and thoughts. The very emotions we are encouraged to keep at bay lest they interfere with sound decision-making have turned out to be critical to our assignment of priorities and thus to making appropriate choices. According to Dr. Damasio, "Reduction in emotion may constitute an equally important source of irrational behavior."

The Permanence of Fear

B ut of all the emotions engaged in our lives, which ones are the most influential? Fear appears to be a particularly strong emotion, and we often feel the effects of fear in marked physiologic ways. Investigators have perhaps studied fear more than any other emotion, and it appears that memories involving fear are permanently ingrained in the brain. Phobias may then be attributed to some dysfunction of the amygdala, which help modify emotions in the brains. These small structures located deep within the brain on both sides help establish memories of events and record the emotional content of those memories, again in neurosignatures or notes that enable the brain to recall the patterns of nerve cell activity associated with the initial incidents.

Fear appears to be a major contributor to the mysterious sudden-death phenomenon among Hmong refugees, members of the Laotian ethnic group who fled Southeast Asia for the United States during the Vietnam War. Sudden unexpected nocturnal death syndrome (SUNDS) is alarmingly common among male Hmong refugees between twenty-five and forty-four years of age, affecting 92 per 100,000 Hmong men. To give you a comparison, these figures would make it the fifth leading cause of natural death in the U.S. male population. Victims appear to die from rare disturbances in cardiac electrical conduction, which occur during their sleep, but autopsies have revealed no structural heart abnormalities. Most of the deaths occur among male refugees who have been in the United States two years or less; the phenomenon does not exist in Laos.

I pause to tell you that I do not mean to frighten you by using extreme examples of the nocebo effect such as SUNDS and voodoo death. Instead I am trying to show the extent to which the mind can affect the body. Later in the book, I'll tell you about the other end of the spectrum—the positive extremes of healing, affirmative beliefs.

Returning for now to our discussion of SUNDS, Dr. Shelley Adler of the University of California, San Francisco, has studied the syndrome in the context of the Hmong culture and concludes that an emotional reaction like no other, a fierce combination of "fear, awe and abasement," causes "cataclysmic psychological distress" that results in sudden death. What causes this unusual but very real fear? Men who have been revived from SUNDS-related cardiac arrests describe having experienced a horrific nightmare, not just your average bad dream but a specific and extreme version they call *tsog tsuam*. Well recognized in their culture, *tsog tsuam* is an evil spirit that visits its victim during the night, sitting on a person's chest and making it difficult to breathe, eventually suffocating him or her.

Chia, one of the patients Dr. Adler interviewed, was very worried about his family and his livelihood during the initial months of being in the United States. He recalls:

I remember a few months after I first came here—I was asleep. I turned out the light and everything, but

I kind of think about, think about, think about, and
then—all of a sudden, I felt that—I cannot move. I
just feel it, but I don't see anything, but I—then I
tried to move my hand, but I cannot move my hand.
I keep trying, but I cannot move myself. I know it is
tsog tsuam. I am so scared. I can hardly breathe. I
think, "Who will help me? What if I die?"

Dr. Adler believes that the men gripped with SUNDS are in
the midst of particularly vulnerable stages of their lives. They
are usually depressed about being unable to uphold the traditional expectations of men in Hmong households since coming to the United States. Their wives and children may have
begun to usurp some of the power and prominence Hmong
men typically enjoy at home, and the men often feel less capable of protecting their families from evil spirits and invaders,
because American society discourages their traditional use of
shamans or religious sacrificial rites.

Of course this is an extreme example, but, when exacerbated by a sense of powerlessness, fear can be a very strong
emotion with severe physical repercussions. Fear appears to
make a particular impression on the brain's amygdala, the
physical significance of which can be reduced over time but
never banished entirely unless the amygdala is damaged. Researchers have studied amygdala damage in rats and found
that in these cases, the animals did indeed forget to be afraid.
Dr. Damasio and scores of other investigators have witnessed
similar reactions in stroke, accident, and other patients who
sustained injuries to specific areas of their brains. Depending
on the injury, these victims experience personality changes,
some dramatic in scope, so that families and colleagues, as
well as the patients themselves, have difficulty adjusting to the
new "self." People with bilateral damage to the amygdala become fearless; they walk alone late at night without considering that it might be dangerous and they get themselves into
all kinds of trouble.

Remembered Wellness and Emotion

W hy is it important that we understand the role of fear and other emotions? Because remembered wellness is an emotionally charged memory, as are voodoo death and other examples of the nocebo effect. When we receive a diagnosis or a clean bill of health, our brains attach certain values to this news. And as it turns out, what we feel about the news may be far more important to the body's dispatch of signals about our health than an objective fact. When we hear about cancer survival rates, they may not register as strong an impression in our brains as the memory we have of a friend who lost all her hair and got very weak but eventually banished cancer from her body.

The vast conglomeration of nerve cells in the amygdala and other regions retains all sorts of memories and assigns emotions to those events based on the enormous history of life influences and experiences to which you have been exposed. If your contacts with the medical profession have been positive, you are apt to assign positive emotional reactions to receiving medical care, and the nerve cells involved in your neurosignature interact with other nerve cells in the brain to pass on and record their positive reading of the event. If on the other hand, in the case of voodoo, you are cursed by a witch doctor in whom you and the people in the village in which you have lived all your life have placed total faith, your fear may tragically trigger other neurosignatures to bring on sudden death.

Dr. Stephen M. Oppenheimer at the Johns Hopkins University Medical School has identified a small spot in the brain called the insular cortex that may be responsible for the sudden deaths often attributed to extreme fright, as happens in voodoo and crime victim deaths, and to those who are said to have died from "broken hearts." When activated by either extreme despair or panic, the insular cortex appears to cause heart damage, just as it does in people who suffer from a life-threatening heartbeat irregularity called ventricular fibrillation. With these two insights—the fact that top-down or thought-induced events are possible and that emotions work in the brain to assign priorities to events that are stored and recalled in neurosignatures—we may begin to understand the potential of remembered wellness and, conversely, of the no-cebo effect.

Wiring and the Will to Live

Another important component in our understanding of remembered wellness, however, is the brain's ultimate priority, established in us even before we are born. This priority is to survive, the propensity for which we call "the will to live." We come into the world with some factory-installed elements, with some neurosignatures already instilled in our brains. This inborn wiring gives the body the guidelines it needs to thrive, to ensure blood and oxygen flow, immune system functioning, our perception of sights and sounds, and other basic survival mechanisms. This wiring is determined by our genes, by the contributions of the egg and sperm at the moment of our conception.

One of the specifics with which we are born is a fear of heights. In one example, infants have been placed on sheets of see-through plexiglass that are secured to the top of a dark table. Even though the plexiglass pane extends beyond the table on both sides and there are no perceivable tactile differences on the pane, the infants who are called to by their mothers will not crawl beyond the confines of the tabletop. They inherently understand the danger of the drop-off they perceive, even though the drop-off does not actually exist.

Among humans, the fear of snakes is almost as universal as the fear of heights. I am no stranger to this phenomenon. One autumn I planted tulip bulbs in the backyard only to be foiled by squirrels who kept digging them up. To frighten and deter the squirrels, I bought a six-foot inflatable plastic snake that, when positioned near the tulip bed, did the trick. But the next spring, after layers of snow had melted, leaving only layers of autumn leaves, I was raking the yard and unearthed my fake snake. Though it was a harmless impostor, it scared the living daylights out of me, and I shouted and leapt backward, only to be relieved that no one had seen me.

I owe this embarrassment to what some researchers call "hard wiring"—the traits with which we are born that seek to ensure survival. Scientists have argued for decades about whether the fear of snakes is hard-wired or learned in life. Dr. Charles Pellegrino, an archaeologist and anthropologist, maintains that our fear of snakes is inborn, dating back to human mammal ancestors of 65 to 100 million years ago. These small mammals' major predators were huge snakes. According to Dr. Pellegrino, it is this innate fear that makes snake and dragon folklore common in so many different cultures.

Of course, psychiatrist Dr. Sigmund Freud suggested that snakes are phallic symbols and that our fears might be sexual in nature. But revisiting the debate in 1979, Dr. Edward J. Murray and Dr. Frank Foote of the University of Miami Department of Psychology issued a questionnaire to sixty college students to gauge their fear of snakes, their actual experiences with snakes, and the conditioning they received about snakes (e.g., reading about or seeing films of snake attacks or witnessing fear of snakes in others). Drs. Murray and Foote learned that the greater the number of direct experiences the study participants had had with snakes, the less apt they were to fear the reptiles. And vice versa, the participants who had little or no direct experiences with snakes—the vast majority of the group—exhibited great fear of them.

Because the phobia was so prevalent and so rarely confirmed in reality, the investigators suggested that "a preparedness for developing a fear of snakes" exists among humans. We can speculate, as does Dr. Pellegrino, that because of the threat snakes posed for our distant ancestors, the brain is hard-wired with the fear of snakes. As we have evolved, living in areas in which snakes represent less of a threat and reassured by the existence of venom kits, perhaps this neural instinct has diminished, leaving a less clear-cut impression. Nevertheless, this impression is easily manipulated and these fears are cultivated and promulgated in storytelling.

The Fight-or-Flight Response Revisited

The fight-or-flight response also appears to be hard-wired. Nobel Prize–winner Dr. Walter R. Hess demonstrated that the fight-or-flight response was evoked by the stimulation of a portion of the brain, a discovery made in animals that is true in humans as well. We inherited from earlier generations the physiologic ability to fight effectively or run away from danger because our ancestors were unlikely to survive without it. Similar to the fear of snakes, even though our experiences of life may differ from those who came before us, we retain a genetic wisdom of the ages, designed to secure our future on earth.

We've long known that genes determine eye color and gender. And in what are sometimes unsettling revelations, science is rapidly identifying genes that make individuals and families vulnerable to certain cancers and diseases. But lately, genetic research has begun to assign predispositions in ways that seem to threaten our very notion of free will, suggesting that everything from sexual orientation to obesity, alcoholism to intelligence is biologically determined. We fear heights and snakes because our genes told us to do so. We have violent tendencies, some scientists have suggested, because of a deficiency of serotonin. Some of the differences between the sexes result from different ways in which men and women use their brains. And human emotions, personalities, even eccentricities and quirks appear to be nothing but the everyday excretions of an organism.

But lest you think that biology rules, that nature conquers nurture in that tired debate, here's a remarkable truth. The brain is malleable and changes constantly, millisecond after millisecond, according to our life experiences. Even though we are born with a set of instructions and neurosignatures, our brains perpetually recruit new nerve cells and nerve-cell-activation patterns to handle its daily inputs—the cereal you eat at breakfast, a smile from your newborn, your rainy commute, and the deadlines and quotas expected of you at work. The minutiae of our lives are always absorbed and evaluated, our brains modifying themselves to handle whatever threats our lifestyles entail.

So not only is the brain the world's most efficient repository, a chronicler and librarian the efficiency and speed of which has yet to be even remotely mimicked by any computer; not only is the brain a trampoline from which springs all action and thought; not only are you endowed from the day you are born with survival instincts; but the brain is its own artist, its own chemist and engineer, constantly remaking and reconstituting itself. You are, at this very moment, a very different organism from the one you were seconds ago and the one you will be seconds from now. The decision-making structures of your brain direct all this traffic, not only relying on tried-and-true routes of nerve cell activation but designing new combinations of nerve cells and neurotransmitters to aid your survival and to help you learn new things.

Brain Plasticity

Scientists call this capacity for change "plasticity." A recent study demonstrated that rats raised in cages that featured toys and mazes grew more neural connections than did rats in empty cages. And thanks to brain plasticity, the same is true in humans. Drs. Avi Karni and Leslie Underleider of the National Institute of Mental Health conducted an experiment in which participants were asked to practice an exercise for ten minutes every day for several weeks: tapping their fingers sequentially—index finger to pinkie—on their thumb. The participants got quite good at it, doubling their speed and accuracy over the course of the four-week study. Periodically, the volunteers performed the finger-to-thumb exercise while having their brains scanned—this time by way of functional magnetic resonance imaging—which enabled the investigators to identify the parts of the brain being used. Each time they received brain scans, the volunteers were also asked to perform the reverse sequence—pinkie to index finger—an activity they had not rehearsed.

On the scans conducted at the very start of the four-week study, Drs. Karni and Underleider found that the original and reversed sequence tasks produced the same-sized areas of activity in the area of the brain called the motor cortex. But after four weeks of rehearsing, the scan taken during the rehearsed sequence revealed an expanded hub of activity in the motor cortex greater than was present in the spontaneously performed task. The investigators concluded that repetition of the task, the frequent convening of particular like-minded nerve cells, recruited other nerve cells in the motor cortex, enlarging and changing the neural connections that were initially involved.

Much like the vocabulary we use to describe our computer hardware and software, our brains have hard wiring and soft wiring. We are hard-wired to fear heights, probably snakes, and anything else that threatened the survival of our forefathers and mothers. We are hard-wired to fight or flee and to rejuvenate ourselves with the relaxation response. But we also have adaptable wiring that enables us to learn new things and to practice new ways of thinking that can, over time, replace the patterns of thinking the brain was accustomed to inputting, evaluating, and acting upon.

All of us have distinct neurosignatures—for wellness, for illness, for strength and endurance, for headaches and nausea, for mobility and pleasure, for pain and disability, for the symptoms you associate with arthritis or angina, and for the specifics you associate with all the other activities and situations you have faced in life. Like a bad habit, or conversely like a good habit, recurring top-down thoughts, along with their corresponding emotional values, engage your brain's previously used nerve-cell-firing patterns to instruct the body. This is how our thoughts become self-fulfilling prophecies, and how our beliefs gear our bodies for the splendid opportunities of remembered wellness.

We cannot yet change our hard-wired genetic predispositions and instincts by behavioral decisions alone, at least not in a time span that we, or our grandchildren, or even our grandchildren's grandchildren would be able to detect. And while genetic engineering may prove possible, the implications and ethics of altering our hard wires are another matter altogether. For now, let's accomplish everything we can by taking advantage of the marvelous malleability of our soft wirings.

When we change our minds, literally and figuratively, we can do a great deal to improve our health. Clearly our bodies and minds are composites of both genetic predispositions and adaptations inspired by our experiences. Nature and nurture are inseparable and interdependent, predestination and free will mingling naturally in our lives. Since both elements determine our neurosignatures—the very wirings of our brains that enable us to contemplate our bodies and our existence—the arguments over the dominance and superiority of either mind or body are ridiculous, their points moot.

Phantom Limbs

There is perhaps no more fascinating example of the interplay between genetic hard wires and the plasticity of the brain than in the experience of amputees. In people who have had hands amputated, one study demonstrates that the part of the brain that once registered sensations in that missing hand vanishes. And yet Dr. Ronald Melzack, a psychologist at McGill University in Montreal, writes in *Scientific American* that 70 percent of amputees report a phenomenon called "phantom limb" sensations—burning, cramping, and shooting pains that they attribute to the absent body part. Other sensations include feeling pressure, warmth or cold, wetness, sweat, itching, ticklishness, and prickliness. The experience is so real to the patients, according to Dr. Melzack, that not only can they vividly describe the sensations and their precise locations, patients will try to lift a cup with a nonexistent hand, or step out of bed with a foot that is not there.

There are a variety of nervous system functions responsible for this phenomenon, which, by the way, also occurs in children born without limbs. Phantom limbs and their pain, according to Dr. Melzack, do fade over time but do not disappear completely, sometimes returning decades after they seem to have gone away. Even if the area of the brain that registered the sensations of the limb vanishes, it's possible that other nerve cells and circuits of the brain retain a memory of the limb. Many brain researchers believe that people are born to—and our brains are hard-wired to—experience limbs. In other words, the very picture that we have of our body, the fact that we have a body at all, is because our brains tell us we do. Or as Dr. Melzack puts it, "We do not need a body to feel a body."

This research promotes a radically different view of the world, a retreat from the idea of the splendidly mechanical body and the diminutive mind that Descartes introduced and society adopted wholeheartedly. The brain produces the experience of the body, not only by interpreting stimuli from both within and outside the body but by generating perceptions on its own, independent of the body and the environment, and thus independent of what we have always thought to be "reality." Dr. Damasio concurs, writing, "We do not know, and it is improbable that we will ever know, what 'absolute' reality is like." He explains, "All that you can know for certain is that [images] are real to your self, and that other beings make comparable images."

Thus, we know ourselves only because the brain exists to tell us who we are, to transfer and interpret signals from the world at large, signals from the body, and signals from our thoughts and imaginations. And our brains consider all these components "real" and important, our emotions and imaginings no less vital than our blood flow and our sense of touch.

Within us is a system of checks and balances in which the hard wires "know" enough to let the soft wires adapt to one's daily and lifelong experiences. At the same time, however, acting as a parent would with a child, the hard wires exert influence over the malleable circuits, setting basic guidelines that must be maintained for survival. It's uncanny to think that this rapid and everybody-talking-at-once dialogue goes on inside of us, shaping and determining our fate, physiologically as we are accustomed to thinking of it, and completely as the new brain research encourages us to appreciate.

It is possible to mobilize our thoughts to change the way our brains work, to shape our nerve cells with experiences and events that are emotionally fulfilling and not emotionally threatening, and to take full advantage of the newly discovered power of top-down or thought-induced brain functions. This is remembered wellness, the potential of which seems boundless when we realize that we can markedly control brain activity, that we can assign priorities to diagnoses and medicines, and that we can rehearse affirmations, visualizations, and other exercises to expand the hotbeds of nerve cells that fire off signals to our hearts, lungs, and limbs.

What stands in our way? Only a stodgy dichotomy separating mind from matter, only an accepted system, which this accumulation of brain research will eventually topple. The medical system is in crisis, as we'll see in the upcoming chapter. And the best remedy of all may lie in the promise of remembered wellness, and in the yet untapped resources that our brilliant brains and visceral souls make possible.

CHAPTER 5

MEDICINE'S SPIRITUAL CRISIS

The pace of change in Western medicine is staggering. There are, at last count, more than 3,500 medical journals in the world, which weekly and monthly besiege physicians and researchers with new findings—the identification of a gene for obesity, the trial of a combination of drugs that researchers hope will delay the onset of full-blown AIDS, theories about how men and women use their brains differently, and steps toward a better understanding of breast cancer. Moreover, doctors have to deal with nonscientific changes—the upheaval in U.S. health care financing, cutbacks in personnel and resources, and restructuring of hospitals and hospital alliances.

Since insurers began instituting strict limits on hospital stays, hospitals have relinquished healthier patients in less precarious medical situations to outpatient surgery and other quick-service clinics. Teaching hospitals, such as the Deaconess Hospital in Boston where I work, care for much sicker patients who require much more intensive or hazardous treatment than did patient populations of teaching hospitals in the past. And while the pace may be exaggerated on Dr. Michael Crichton's TV version, ER, the demands on caregivers to keep up with breakthroughs and setbacks, with economic forecasts and paperwork requirements, with "code blues" and needlestick precautions, with fast-moving gurneys and insurer limits, are colossal. And I'm afraid that the things that imbue our patients' lives with meaning—the values, fears, and sources of solace that immediately come to mind when one's health is threatened—frequently get disregarded in this whirlwind of change.

My quest for something longer lasting is, in part, a reaction to this medical system and its turmoil. On both a macro, systemic level and on a personal level, I feel the influence individuals and their minds, emotions, and beliefs can have over their healing is being neglected. This has long been true. After all, I had had a very difficult time in the 1960s persuading my colleagues that stress could be a contributor to high blood pressure as I had shown in some of my early experiments with monkeys. And in 1968, when I brought practitioners of Transcendental Meditation into the laboratory to study the physiology of meditation, several of my mentors recommended that I put aside any further exploration of TM. They told me I was throwing away a promising career.

I have come to believe that this depreciation of the power of the patient is a symptom of a larger crisis in American medicine. And to alleviate it, I had to appreciate the factors contributing to the malaise both health care professionals and patients were experiencing. I've outlined the symptoms and problems first, and then traced the history of mind/body effects in medicine. You'll see how medicine came to dismiss a wonderful faculty of human physiology that I believe may bring better health to both the medical system and to patients themselves.

A Privileged Position

From the start, however, I must point out that we evaluate and critique the American medical community from a position of tremendous privilege, because most of our citizens have access to far better treatment and care than most of the world's citizens. Whatever criticisms one might have of the current American health care system, we still enjoy the most advanced, most admired medical care in the world.

I can vouch for that myself because three years ago on Halloween, I had an accident that nearly took my life. I was at home and had just covered the ceiling air-conditioning vents with plastic to prevent the cold drafts that come with the long New England winter. I was on my way to take a shower when I noticed a corner of plastic that had not adhered to the vent in the kitchen. Foolishly, I mounted a chair that slides in and out from the table by way of metal runners. Before I could fix the plastic, the chair slid out from under me, shooting me backward like a missile. I fell, hitting the back of my rib cage on the long end of a butcher block table. As it turns out, I broke five ribs and punctured a lung, causing the lung to collapse and the right side of my chest to fill with blood and other fluids.

Hearing the racket, my wife came quickly and found me lying on the floor in agony, only able to take shallow breaths. She dialed 911, paramedics arrived promptly, and I was transported to the emergency room of the nearby Lahey Clinic, where surgeons inserted a tube into my chest that expanded the collapsed lung and sucked out the fluids that had accumulated. My healthy breathing was restored, although I had a lengthy recovery ahead of me due to my broken ribs.

I will briefly digress to tell you that as the paramedics carried me down the front steps of our home, I felt the need, as is my predilection, to try to make light of this horrible event. The pain was so great at that point, I rasped to my concerned wife, "This is much worse than childbirth!" The mother of our two children looked at me with somewhat less compassion and retorted, "How would you know?" With that, my hopes of having the last word in this repartee between the sexes were dashed, and I limited myself to unintelligible moans and groans the rest of the way to the hospital.

I tell this story for two reasons. First, having done a really foolish thing that could have cost me my life, I felt a special urgency to write this book and to share what I know about remembered wellness. Secondly, some people might suggest that it was this sparring with my wife that helped distract me from my fear in this terrifying situation. But the truth is, no form of remembered wellness could have revived the function of my lung and saved my life. I needed the tools of modern medicine to breathe properly. There was no substitute.

We take for granted that trauma centers routinely snatch patients from the clutches of death, that diagnostic and screening tests give us months and even years of notice to halt an encroaching disease, and that antibiotics and vaccines save us from scourges that imperiled our ancestors and that continue to imperil much of the world today. Thanks to medicine's marvels, the average life expectancy for Americans is much longer than that enjoyed by previous generations. On the average, white women live to be 79.6, black women to 73.8, white men to 72.9, and black men to 64.6. Yet with the quantity of our years assured, we look to medicine to say more to us about the quality of our lives, and we're disappointed that it so often neglects our "souls."

Like a god that has proven less than divine, medicine's power is becoming suspect. The pharmaceuticals and technologies we hoped would shield us from all of life's terrible facts have failed, at least in the case of many cancers, AIDS, and other so-far-impenetrable scourges. Red and pink ribbons populate our lapels, reminders that we have not conquered all illness, as science once seemed to assure us we would.

Even success comes back to haunt us. Common bacteria have developed resistance to antibiotic therapies, mutating to dodge our magic bullets. As Dr. Mitchell Cohen of the Centers for Disease Control and Prevention recently noted, drug-resistant bacteria already exist in hospitals, nursing homes, and to some degree among the general public, causing infection of surgical wounds and the urinary and respiratory tracts. He says, "The problem [can] become very, very serious. . . . We already have some untreatable infections and some bacteria strains are just an antibiotic away from being untreatable."

Giant Reversals

Medicine is also famous for its flip-flops. Once doctors were confident that a low-roughage diet was the best treatment for an inflammation of the colon called diverticulitis, but a few decades later they urged sufferers instead to eat plenty of roughage. Once, physicians assured postmenopausal women that hormone replacement therapy did not increase likelihood of breast cancer; recently, they have announced the opposite finding. *New England Journal of Medicine* editors Dr. Marcia Angell and Dr. Jerome Kassirer have acknowledged the problem, asking, "What Should the Public Believe?" Health-conscious Americans, the editors say, "increasingly find themselves beset by contradictory advice. No sooner do they learn the results of one study than they hear of one with the opposite message." While Drs. Angell and Kassirer blame the press and public for "unrealistic expectations" of medical science, epidemiologists interviewed in the July 14, 1995, *Science* suggest that epidemiologic studies have inherent drawbacks. The *Science* article's headline and subhead spell out the problem: "Epidemiology Faces Its Limits: The Search for Subtle Links Between Diet, Lifestyle, or Environmental Factors and Disease Is an Unending Source of Fear—But Often Yields Little Certainty."

As science acquires new knowledge, we expect shifts in prevention, diagnosis, and treatment. Lately, however, we've been seeing 180 degree, about-face turns. Combine this with the fact that medicine is practiced quite differently even within the Western world—U.S. doctors, for example, recommend far more hysterectomies and heart-bypass operations than their European counterparts—and we reach a disturbing conclusion: Medicine is less scientific than we've always counted on it to be. A June 25, 1995, *New York Times* article went so far as to say that society's assumption that medical styles are supported by irrefutable evidence "is so far off the mark that the term 'medical science' is practically an oxymoron." One researcher, Dr. David Eddy of the Jackson Hole Group, estimates that no more than 15 percent of medical treatments are founded on "reliable scientific evidence."

The evidence is, in fact, markedly influenced by culture, personal bias and experience, and emotions. Part of the reason experiments contradict one another is because we cannot control for all the different beliefs and expectations individuals bring to these studies. As I have suggested before, if medicine looked for and controlled for commonalties rather than universality, that is, if it allowed for different groups of different minds to produce different results, as diverse people do, science might achieve more consistent results.

Human Error

Like all human endeavors, medicine is also susceptible to human error. Medicine's dictum "First, do no harm" is undermined by the fact that 180,000 hospitalized Ameri-

cans die each year because of errors made by hospital personnel, according to former surgeon Dr. Lucian L. Leape of the
Harvard School of Public Health in the December 1994 *Journal
of the American Medical Association* (*JAMA*). This is the equivalent
of three jumbo-jet crashes every two days. The public is aghast
to hear cases in which a wrong leg is amputated or a toxic dose
of medicine is dispensed, tragic errors in which whole teams of
health care workers are involved. And Dr. Leape's six-month examination of drug prescription and administration in Boston
hospitals published in *JAMA* in July 1995 revealed 334 errors—
one in every fifteen patients—39 percent of which were made
by the doctors ordering drugs, 38 percent by nurses dispensing
them, the rest by secretaries transcribing orders or pharmacists
preparing medications. While most of the errors were caught or
didn't harm anyone, the evidence nevertheless compels medicine to better control quality.

Even more distressing, however, is the fact that the medical
profession maintains an "ostrichlike attitude" about its mistakes, says Dr. David Blumenthal, MPP, associate professor of
medicine at Harvard Medical School. "Mistakes have been
treated as uncommon and atypical, requiring no remedy beyond
the traditional incident reports and morbidity and mortality conferences," Dr. Blumenthal writes in the aforementioned 1994 issue of *JAMA*.

The ostrichlike attitude is not new. As *New York Times* medical writer Dr. Lawrence K. Altman noted recently in response
to a spate of highly publicized medical errors, "Nearly a century ago in Boston, Dr. Ernst A. Codman proposed measuring
the effectiveness of medical care by sending postcards to patients a year after their discharge from the Massachusetts General Hospital. His colleagues saw the pioneering proposal as a
threat, and Dr. Codman, a wealthy Brahmin, had to start his
own hospital."

Morbidity and mortality conferences and autopsies have
long served as physicians' primary gauges of quality control. In
these settings, doctors explain to other doctors how treatment
failed, reviewing pathology reports and, in the case of death, au-
topsy results, to learn from mistakes and improve care. Simul-

taneously but separately, hospital administrators have surveyed patients about the cleanliness of rooms, the food, ease of admission and discharge, and friendliness of staff. Despite the fact that evidence has long existed that satisfied patients heal faster, experience fewer complications, and are discharged sooner, rates of disease and death and those of patient satisfaction have rarely been compared in hospital settings.

Other service industries have long understood that customer relations are as important as first-class products. But medicine has always believed that the problems it solves—injury or illness—supersede all other concerns. If you should find yourself bleeding profusely after a car accident, you'll care far more about the speed and skill of the emergency room staff than about ambiance and cheerfulness. Patients facing cancer treatment want compassion but they'll accommodate a gruff reply far more often if it comes from the leading specialist in the field.

Disenchanted Patients and Doctors

The vast majority of patients—those who seek routine medical care—seem to want better relationships with their physicians. And not surprisingly, doctors want the same thing, especially the time to develop a healing trust. Three-fourths of American doctors say that the pressure of their jobs keeps them from spending enough time with their patients. Imagine spending eight to thirteen years in medical school and training, incurring tens of thousands of dollars in school debt in the process, only to find yourself restricted in the thing you most wanted to do—take proper care of patients. Consider that the partnership physicians want to cultivate with patients is often overseen by a third party, the HMO, insurance company, or another payer, imposing limits on the time doctors have to listen, and demanding that the topic of doctor/patient conversation have an appropriate billing category and code.

As painful as hard economic times have been for hospitals, some good things have come of the ferocious economic competition. Health care facilities have been forced to question and refine their methods in unprecedented ways. Medical departments, not just public or customer relations departments, have recently begun to pursue patient satisfaction with greater seriousness. A July 24, 1995, *New York Times* article reveals that hospitals are adopting the niceties usually associated with hotels. Some New York hospitals are going so far as to send fruit baskets and champagne to new mothers and fathers, and offering high tea and live piano music in their atriums.

"We sometimes get lost in the trenches and forget how we look and appear to the outside world," says Lorraine Tredge, the executive director of North Central Bronx Hospital, which is trying to upgrade its customer service. "We don't even know how to answer our phones. We're way too brusque. Instead of 'North Central Bronx,' it should be 'North Central Bronx. How can I help you?' A small change like that can make a big difference in how we are perceived."

At the same time, health care's escalating costs force impossible choices upon the medical profession and the nation, namely, "How do we withhold expensive treatments from a nation that feels entitled to them?" and "How do we cut services that we know make for better-quality patient care?" In human terms, these questions are devastatingly difficult. Does an elderly woman really need a hip replacement operation? Does an alcoholic patient deserve a liver transplant? Should we save money upfront and send mothers home quickly after they've delivered even if it means greater strain, less time to bond with and learn about the newborn, and greater risk of infant death due to unrecognized and untreated dehydration and jaundice? In general, can the health care system afford to let patients spend less time developing good relationships with caregivers?

A Spiritual Crisis

Author John Updike once observed that America is not a victim of limits, but of dreams: "There is no enough. That's one of the words Americans have a very hard time learning: the word enough." This is at the heart of medicine's quandary, in which both health care professionals and patients vacillate between bitter denial and the glare of the 1990s—the painful acknowledgment of exorbitant price tags, human frailties, and the limits that hem in our dreams.

This is a spiritual crisis. The god of science we once believed had the power to stamp out disease and delay death's eventual toll is proving inadequate. Scientific medicine may have transformed and reconfigured hope for our ancestors, amazed as they were that human intelligence and scientific methods could wrest from God what was previously considered a divine decision—who would live and who would die. But the discoveries that once inspired awe are now taken for granted in society. And perhaps most frustrating of all, medicine has confined its definitions of "what we are made of" to cells and bones, not the rich gamut of moods and ideas, passions and values that we feel in our bones must be, to a certain extent, organically controlled.

History Reviewed

I t wasn't always this way. In fact, throughout history, medicine had to rely on the human spirit and other seemingly mysterious sources of miracles. Let's face it, in the beginning, there was the placebo. And for primitive medicine, the placebo was all there was. Early medicine and its cross-cultural cast of characters—priests, healers, sorcerers, medicine men, witch doctors, witches, shamans, midwives, herbalists, physicians, and surgeons—relied exclusively on scientifically unproved potions and procedures, the vast majority of which had no physical value in and of themselves, some of which did more harm than good. The fact that some patients got better had much more to do with the natural course of their diseases or illness and with the power of belief than with the inherent value of the medicine.

Placebo effect expert Dr. Arthur K. Shapiro of Mount Sinai School of Medicine noted that before the advent of scientific medicine in the twentieth century patients endured "purging, puking, poisoning, cutting, cupping, blistering, bleeding, freezing, heating, sweating, leeching and shocking" and were advised to consume "lizard's blood, crocodile dung, pig's teeth, putrid meat, fly specks, frog's sperm, powdered stone, human sweat, worms, spiders, furs, and feathers." Almost all human and animal excretions were consumed or applied in medical treatments, as was moss scraped from the skull of a person who had been hanged. Generations of those who cringed before they swallowed are perhaps the source of an expression we use today, namely, "If it tastes this bad, it's got to be good for you."

People underwent treatments that today we'd call out-landish. Tattoos were applied over the areas of pain. Discov-ered in the Tyrolean Alps in 1991, the five-thousand-year-old remains of the so-called Ice Man had tattoo markings on his calf and lower legs over places where, X-rays revealed, he had had osteoarthritis. According to Dr. Torstein Sjovoid of the University of Stockholm, these tattoos were made of soot and carved into the skin.

Until recently, medicine and superstition were closely tied. There was an aura and mystery to what were essentially placebo treatments. As documented by University of California profes-sor Wayland D. Hand in his comprehensive book *Magical Med-icine*, "passing through" rituals were common in primitive medicine. To help patients "go through" and emerge on the other side of illness, healers passed infants through wedged openings in trees, or pulled people through holes in rocks or through tunnels in the earth. Intersections of roads were con-sidered important healing sites, so patients were urged to rub salt on themselves, to throw gravel, or to leave some of their fin-gernails to deposit disease at a crossroads. To cure malaria, a pa-tient had to walk three times around a pot that had a toad under it; for some eye maladies, a patient would be adminis-tered urine from a "faithful wife." An arthritic patient was di-rected to find yarn spun by a girl under seven years of age. The midnight hour was always attributed with special power, and people were encouraged to fetch water for healing and to pluck medicinal herbs from the ground at that late hour.

Because these superstitions and legends were accepted and touted by healers, they undoubtedly fostered remembered wellness. And up until about a hundred years ago, remembered wellness was the treatment of choice. Some of the early herbal remedies, perhaps as many as 25 to 50 percent, contained active agents that might have contributed to healing, maintains the noted medical historian Dr. Erwin H. Ackerknecht. However, because those herbs were prescribed widely and randomly, for vastly different diseases and ailments, it is unlikely the active ingredients were applied in ways in which healing could occur. Moreover, active ingredients were often compromised in poor preparation, lack of refrigeration, and in combination with toxic ingredients.

Acupuncture, so often cited as an ancient treatment with modern merit, may have done more harm than good in its history. Practiced in China for more than 2,500 years, acupuncture has been shown by Western medicine to be effective in relieving some kinds of pain and in easing the symptoms of withdrawal from drug addiction—results I predict will eventually be largely attributed to remembered wellness. But because acupuncture was performed with unsterile needles for most of those 2,500 years, it also undoubtedly contributed to China's hepatitis epidemics.

Medicine Equaled the Placebo Effect

In large measure, the history of medicine is the history of the placebo effect. Well into the twentieth century, despite the influence science had begun to wield in other realms of the world at that time, medicine still offered more care than it did cures, more attention than technology. Ironically, the reputation physicians have enjoyed throughout history, privileged and esteemed in every culture and time one can name, was built on and cultivated by the success of remembered wellness and on the three modes of belief-inspired healing: the belief of an individual in a treatment, the belief of the caregiver, or their mutual beliefs.

Recognizing this trend, Galen the Greek physician, born around A.D. 130, is attributed with saying, "He cures most in whom most are confident." In early medicine and in cultures that resist the influence of Western scientific medicine, maintaining their own traditions, the relationship between healer and patient is sacred and mystical in quality. The African medicine man wears special garb, offers incantations, and observes certain rituals, all of which lend the delivery of medicine a special aura and importance, greater than pills and procedures, seemingly connected in more substantial ways to the world around them. Josiah Gregg, a Santa Fe trader, encountered Comanche Indians in the 1840s and took note of the intense faith they had in their tribal medicine men. Gregg observed that a patient's imagination was often called upon in rituals that seemed to hasten recovery. Scientific verification or no, the Indian tradition, in which repetitive singing was used to ward off disease-bearing demons, appeared to work on a patient's behalf.

The Shona people of Rhodesia have traditionally sought help from a healer known as a *nganga*. The mutual esteem, affection, and sympathy between patient and healer, as reported by Dr. Michael Gelfand, who practiced medicine in South Africa for many years, sets their tradition apart from the sterile, rushed delivery of medicine we, alas, have come to expect in the West.

Seneca, the Latin philosopher who lived from about 4 B.C. to A.D. 65, appreciated the role of hope, saying, "It is part of the cure to wish to be cured." After all, for most of recorded history, individuals bore responsibility for their own health; people tried to live good lives in order to maintain an equilibrium, a balance of humors—black and yellow bile, blood and phlegm—that ensured health of mind and body. External factors such as climate or environment could upset the balance, but people believed they had the ability to restore the equilibrium. If they could not and disease occurred, the physician was called upon to restore humors to their proper proportions.

Illness as God's Judgment

I n his scholarly book *The Limits of Medicine*, historian Dr. Edward S. Golub writes that for a very long span of human history, illness and infections were believed to occur when one lost favor with God or gods. This sentiment survives in a different form today. Modern society fosters other cause-and-effect views of disease—that the affliction is the result of a virus, a bacterium, a poison, or bad living—too much alcohol, smoking, eating the wrong foods, exercising too little or too much, or not learning to handle stress. Either consciously or subconsciously, many Americans consider it a failure of character when a person succumbs to illness or death. And similarly, physicians consider illness and death "professional failures." Later in the book we will talk about the ravages of guilt that accompany this type of thinking. But for now, suffice it to say that because disease was previously supposed to be the result of some divine judgment, doctors and hospitals were generally considered powerless to interfere if death was indeed God's edict.

Self-diagnosis and medication were the norm. In Europe up until the mid-1800s, the gentry were the only class with access to doctors. Both the rich and the poor relied on elixirs and salves, readily available from street vendors and shopkeepers. But neither the emerging profession of medicine nor the neighbor lady with her stash of home remedies had much power over the blight and death that raged throughout Europe. Up until the twentieth century, a full quarter of children died before their first birthdays, and average life expectancy was thirty years. Working-class people lived in squalor, without baths, drains, or sewage systems and with little or no way to dispose of refuse, animal or human waste, rotting meats and vegetables, or even dead bodies. In 1840, English gentry whose homes had better sanitation lived on average to the ripe old age of forty-three, while laborers typically died at twenty-three.

Sanitation and Science

With the sanitation movement came the first realization by much of the Western world that disease was traceable to a particular source. People stopped blaming illness on shifting humors and the will of God and began to realize that contaminated water and rotten food were really the problem. Sweeping across Europe beginning in the mid-1800s, government-mandated waterworks, sewage systems, burial and waste disposal standards, paved streets, and extensions of health care to the disadvantaged made dramatic gains on scourges like cholera and typhoid fever. In 1853, five years after modest changes in sanitation were implemented in 284 English towns, the death rate of the working class was cut by more than half, dropping from 30 per 1,000 to 13.

More radical change was in store. Science and technology were marching into every aspect of life, steam engines fueling transportation and industry, electricity affording civilization the telegraph and light bulbs. Indeed, the world was starting to make more sense, as forces previously considered mysterious and all-powerful were being tamed and managed. City life was far more organized and strategically planned than farm communities had needed to be. With the Enlightenment, Dr. Golub teaches, people were empowered to "do" rather than to think, to conquer the environment rather than to pray for deliverance from it. Heady with their growing mastery of the elements, people began for the first time to expect cures, not just care.

As they learned that the earth revolved around the sun rather than vice versa, and that a force called gravity kept us weighted in our world, people began to assign names to and explanations for a previously nebulous reality. In the process, the religious beliefs and life meaning that had carried humanity through wars, famines, plagues, and so many inexplicable periods of history began to lose their luster. There was no end to the questions men and women had for their universe, and seemingly no end to the answers in that day. So even though human beliefs and remembered wellness were irrepressible, they became less and less relevant, their effects on the human condition considered unmeasurable and thus insignificant.

The Great Discoveries

For thousands of years medicine relied on remembered wellness, yielding haphazard successes. But overnight it seems, starting with Drs. Louis Pasteur and Robert Koch, the speedometer jumped from 0 to 100 miles per hour and then the pedal stuck. In 1854, the French chemist Louis Pasteur determined that yeast was responsible for making distilled sugar beets ferment into vinegar. Pasteur launched the modern-day germ theory, our understanding of microscopic organisms that live and interact within us. And in 1874, rural German physician Robert Koch identified the bacteria that caused anthrax in sheep. Later, Koch discovered that both tuberculosis and cholera were caused by specific bacteria. Having identified that specific bacteria cause specific diseases, it became the goal of every scientist to specify problems and develop bacteria-counteracting medicines, a far more focused view of the cause and treatment of illness than was prevalent before.

For the first time in history, the role of belief in activating remembered wellness did not seem to matter. If you got a puncture from a rusty nail, you would, as a result of Dr. Emil Behring and Dr. Shibasaburo Kitasato's discovery in 1890, be given a small dose of tetanus bacterium toxin to prevent tetanus or lockjaw. It didn't matter if you believed in the treatment, it didn't matter if the doctor handing the drug to you laughed out loud and uproariously at the prospect of it working, it didn't matter if the relationship between the two of you was hostile and scornful, the treatment worked!

Modern medicine came to expect that all healing could be accomplished with specific medications. A god or spirit no longer needed to be invoked, because humanity on its own, with the discovery of vitamins, was eradicating the scourges of scurvy, beriberi, pellagra, and rickets. Juvenile diabetics, many of whom never lived long enough to become adults, could, thanks to the discovery of insulin by Sir Frederick G. Banting, Dr. Charles H. Best, and Dr. John J.R. Macleod in Toronto in 1922, be kept alive and well with daily injections.

In 1929, Sir Alexander Fleming took a holiday from his work at St. Mary's Hospital in London but upon returning to the petri dishes he had left in his laboratory found that they were covered with bacteria growth. However, where bread mold had grown, the bacteria had not. From this observation, Fleming discovered that bread mold produced penicillin.

In those days, half of all adults over fifty contracted and died from pneumonia. Dr. Maxwell Finland, one of my teachers at Harvard, was practicing at the Boston City Hospital in the late 1930s when Dr. Fleming's brainchild was introduced onto the medical wards. Dr. Finland tried to communicate to us—so unimaginable was a world without antibiotics to me and my medical school classmates—the metamorphosis that occurred in his own thinking when patients of his, whom he expected to die overnight from pneumonia, were up and around the next day, eating and chatting, after a single dose of penicillin. So expensive and rare was penicillin at that time that the staff collected patients' urine, boiled it and gave it to other patients to drink so those patients would be cured of pneumonia as well.

Since antiquity, health had been a mysterious matter—illness brought on by a strange shifting of intangible internal forces. Healers were humbled in the face of fate, leaving recovery in the hands of God or the individual. But in the twentieth century, scientific medicine produced so-called miracles as if on an assembly line. As promised in the Bible, the blind were made to see, only not by faith but by cataract surgery.

Removing the Constant Threat

When science and sanitation first began to thwart disease and death, it transformed people's everyday experiences and their whole worldview. Dr. Golub says that even in his great-grandparents' time, death was associated with youth, and if a person lived to old age, he or she had lost many contemporaries along the arduous journey. He reminds us that for many, many years, birth and marriage were far less striking features of family life than was "the constant presence of death." With cemeteries at the center of town, death was the central reality of people's lives.

Of all the changes science introduced by the start of the twentieth century—electric lights, transportation, photography, hot-air balloons, telegraphs, phonographs, moving pictures, and X-rays—Dr. Golub says that the most important in the mind of the public was that science "eliminated the constant presence of death." It delivered people from a previously unrelenting onslaught of images, odors, and sounds of suffering and death. As a result, he writes, the public began idolizing scientists, deferring to them as if they were miracleworkers. "Their children could be saved from dying of diphtheria; the causes of tuberculosis, cholera, typhoid and syphilis were known; surgery was now safer; and the constant presence of death was becoming a memory only of the old people."

Nevertheless, well into the twentieth century, medicine maintained some of the views that had dominated science during "the constant death" era. Historian Charles Rosenberg describes the prevailing medical model of the late nineteenth and early twentieth century as "all-inclusive, anti-reductionistic, capable of incorporating every aspect of man's life in explaining his physical condition." Disease was still treated as if it were a natural imbalance, an interaction of biological, behavioral, moral, psychological, and spiritual factors.

Doctors often prescribed multifaceted regimens including medications, special diets, behavior modifications, and changes of location—regimens that were supposed to reflect an intimate knowledge of the patient's personal and family idiosyncrasies. Dr. Rosenberg writes, "No mid-19th century physician doubted the efficacy of placebos (as little as he doubted the effectiveness of a drug could depend on his own manner and attitude)." And Dr. Richard C. Cabot of the Massachusetts General Hospital

wrote of his nineteenth-century Harvard Medical School education: "Now I was brought up, as I suppose every physician is,
to use what are called placebos, that is bread pills, subcuta-
neous injections of a few drops of water (supposed by the patient to be morphine), and other devices, for acting upon a
patient's symptoms through his mind."

The Rise of Technology

Nevertheless, remembered wellness was gradually
falling out of favor. As my colleague Dr. Samuel S. Myers and I wrote in our 1992 paper, disease was, more
and more, being defined in medicine and in the world not as
an unnatural imbalance but as a deviance from a norm char-
acterized by a growing number of specific, measurable, physiological parameters. Reductionism made heroes of laboratory
scientists such as Drs. Koch and Pasteur, the body becoming a
sum of its increasingly small and complicated parts. Medical
science concerned itself with applying universal truths to treat
individuals rather than focusing on the individual's particular-
ities. And, for many diseases for which a specific cause and
treatment could be identified, this approach was marvelously
successful.

Official condemnations of the use of remembered wellness
quickly followed. In 1910, the Flexner Report was issued. Allopathic medicine, the forefather of current Western medicine,
adopted the Flexner Report, which mandated that only medical
schools that taught scientific medicine could produce licensed
physicians. Allopathic medicine, like the other forms of medicine—homeopathy, osteopathy, hydrotherapy, naturopathy—
had been totally dependent on remembered wellness. But by
espousing scientifically based medicine, it differentiated itself
from its competitors and rejected the notion that the mind
might influence the body, claiming instead that all illness could
be traced to single, specific sources. And by the 1930s,
mind/body reactions and remembered wellness had become so
disreputable that the *Index Medicus*, the listing of all published

articles in medical journals, did not contain a single reference to the effect of the mental state on physiology.

The placebo's only legitimate role in medicine was assigned in the 1950s when it became a benchmark by which to measure new drugs and techniques. In other words, if a new drug or procedure were no better than a placebo, the new treatment would be considered a failure. Never mind that placebos were 30 to 90 percent effective; attention was focused on the next, ever stronger or more aggressive therapy, rather than on a mind/body impetus for healing. The placebo effect essentially became, as I noted earlier, pejorative, or "all in your head."

Despite Vietnam and Watergate and all the pointed questions the American public began to put to the "establishment" in the 1960s and 1970s, medicine and its emphasis on specific cures remained largely unassailable. Whether it was turning back disease or sending a man to the moon, science inspired the nation in turbulent times, progress continuing to be a source of pride. But one need only contrast that giant of friendly, personal attention, television's Dr. Marcus Welby, with the frenzy and distraction of doctors on *St. Elsewhere* or with the procedure-manic physicians on *ER* to surmise that as faith in scientific medicine grew, faith in the caring capacity of doctors diminished.

And by following the medical staff, *ER* perpetuates a mentality that is common among doctors and nurses—that triumphs or failures are personal and professional rather than inevitable, natural occurrences in a life span in which people sometimes get sick and recover, and sometimes get sick and die.

The Modern View

But Western society doesn't think that way anymore. Nature can be overcome. And if you've seen the way many patients die in hospitals today, there's sometimes very little that's natural about it. On the contrary, we expect everything of medicine—the miracles and the impossible "saves," the magic bullets, the fast fixes afforded us by technology, specialization, and their accompanying high costs. With an estimated $1 trillion spent on health care in the United States in 1995, it's clear Americans may still want it all as they did in the 1980s, but we haven't the slightest idea how to pay for it all in the 1990s.

Americans have always liked to win. We like to act on and conquer problems, our accomplishments born of taming the wild and subduing enemies. Appropriately then, medicine has adopted military terms—doctors "giving orders" and serving on medicine's "front lines," often using "magic bullets" to turn back "intruders," according to author Susan Sontag in *Illness As Metaphor*. In a study of informed consent in various cultures, Boston University School of Law professors George J. Annas and Frances H. Miller superbly document this American obsession with medical action. They cite nineteenth-century Harvard Medical School professor Dr. Oliver Wendell Holmes, who believed that the American frontier gave birth to our aggressive medical approach, writing:

> How could a people [that] . . . has contrived the Bowie knife and the revolver . . . [that] insists in sending out yachts and horses and boys to outsail, outrun, outfight and checkmate all the rest of creation; how could such a people be content with any but "heroic" practice? What wonder that the stars and stripes wave over doses of ninety grains of sulfate of quinine and that the American eagle screams with delight to see three drachms of calomel given at a single mouthful?

Americans have trouble fathoming that rest, relief from stress, and the indulgence of time can be healing. For example, doctors in Europe send patients to government-financed spas to relax and heal, a practice that's virtually unheard of in the States. Besides, the exhausted guest of an American spa would be offered a regimen of aerobic classes, supervised walks, weight rooms, and gyms, accentuated by low-calorie vegetarian fare, while European spas emphasize sleep and re-laxation and feature fine wines, chocolate, and other luxuries.

Writer Luigi Barzini suggests that Americans are compelled to act because we believe "the main purpose of a man's life is to solve problems." Despite the fact that the body is the grand-est problem-solver there is, quietly and perpetually sustaining life, overcoming billions of obstacles without our conscious imperatives for it to do so, we don't trust it. Instead, we turn to our medicine cabinets. Our doctors' first impulse is to pre-scribe something for us, and we fully expect to emerge from these visits with a prescription in hand.

But at the same time, record numbers of Americans are spending record numbers of their health care dollars on un-conventional healers—chiropractors, acupuncturists, herbal-ists, and others—who they trust will care more about them as individuals than as sums of parts. While some studies show that patients are generally happy with their own doctors, man-aged care, with its provider lists and required numbers of pa-tients a doctor must see each day, makes this relationship between doctor and patient harder to preserve.

The Reluctance of Physicians

And modern American physicians, while adapting to change in every other sphere, have been slow to resur-rect remembered wellness, which patients are telling us they want from traditional medicine. Doctors are loath to ad-mit that the placebo effect contributes to the success of the treatments they recommend or perform, according to Dr. Charles K. Hofling of the College of Medicine, University of Cincinnati, and Dr. Shapiro, whose extensive explorations into the placebo effect we've referred to before. In their stud-ies, doctors said their peers were three times more likely to employ the placebo effect than they were. And specialists usu-ally excluded their specialty treatments when enumerating the powers of the placebo in medicine. Internists believed their medical practices were free of the effects of the placebo, psychologists excluded psychology, psychiatrists excluded psychotherapy and psychoanalysis, and surgeons excluded surgery. Yet, from the evidence compiled here, we know that every specialty and treatment benefits from affirmative beliefs and remembered wellness, and that every treatment is equally vulnerable to the negative repercussions of the nocebo effect.

Why wouldn't a doctor want to claim remembered wellness? Why wouldn't a doctor want to take credit for establishing a therapeutic relationship with patients and instilling confidence in his or her treatments? First of all, they get little credit for doing so by insurers. At the end of your office visit, in order to be reimbursed for the care the doctor dispensed, he or she fills out a form to indicate the diagnoses made and the actions taken. You can imagine that little room is provided on the form for "stomach problems brought on by tension over passing the bar exam" or "general malaise after the death of a friend," nor does the form provide for "remembered wellness" or "time will heal." Secondly, fear of malpractice or fear of not *doing* something demands that they perpetuate the standard, albeit ineffective, practice.

But in other cases, physicians just don't understand the placebo effect, still considering the placebo a scientific anomaly or unscientific. Some underestimate their personal influence over patients and don't appreciate how helpful an honest but optimistic diagnosis can be, or how therapeutic a friendly manner can be. In other cases, egos get in the way as many doctors don't want to admit that they don't know it all and that they can't explain everything.

Too often, I'm afraid, an all-knowing attitude is cultivated in physicians. We doctors are not encouraged to appreciate invisible or somewhat intangible aspects of healing, nor are we well prepared to teach patients to care for themselves. Starting early in medical school and continuing in hospital training, prospective physicians are routinely quizzed in front of peers and more experienced colleagues; every aspiring doctor is stung early and often by the embarrassment of not being able to produce an answer or of not answering correctly. Of course, more progressive medical school curricula and training programs have tried to intervene by focusing more comprehensively on patient case studies rather than rote memory of body parts and diseases. But by and large, the journey to physician-hood is still a perpetual pop quiz. In a race to provide answers quickly and assuredly, these doctors come to value talking over listening, interrupting over quietude, speed over patience, and action over waiting.

Despite the reluctance of physicians to adopt remembered wellness, we are, without a doubt, at a turning point in the history of belief in healing. Clearly the public is ahead of medicine in articulating the void—the lack of regard for human personalities, for the beliefs and priorities we possess as individuals, or for the spiritual quality of life, which often feels more important to people than the physical reality. Medicine must soon attend to this craving for meaning, this demand that health be defined by more than test results and vital signs.

Following this bouncing ball of belief as we have throughout history, it has taken just over 150 years for humanity to come full circle—to abandon and then redeem the beliefs that aided the survival of men and women from the very start. Venerable still, "reason" and science are used in this book to define belief's centrality to physical survival. The scholars and technologies that stole remembered wellness's thunder are the very ones that are restoring it. The meanings we attach to life have often felt unreal, but bigger than life, transcending reality. But all the while, paradoxically, our beliefs were fiddling inside us and, in real ways, enhancing and preserving life.

CHAPTER 6

THE RELAXATION RESPONSE

Y ou'll recall that the reason I took a closer look at remembered wellness in the first place was because I was asked to distinguish it from the bodily calm I termed the relaxation response. While I was, in true reductionistic fashion, able to establish that the relaxation response could work independently and exclusively of remembered wellness, without the impetus of beliefs behind it, I learned that the relaxation response and remembered wellness can intersect in very influential and meaningful ways. In fact, these mechanisms complement each other very well.

In this chapter, I'll introduce you to the relaxation response and its relevance to my increasing fascination with the physical actions of belief on people's health. (You'll find more details about the relaxation response in my book of the same name, *The Relaxation Response*.) You'll see that even though science can divide the relaxation response and belief very easily for the purpose of study, measurements, and replication, patients readily apply their beliefs, values, and meanings to mental focusing techniques. This makes for a very dynamic duo of healing.

At six one Sunday morning several years ago, a neighbor two houses up the street summoned me for help. Paul was a nationally known men's suit designer, his wife, Marie, the backbone of their very close Italian family. We had been neighbors for fifteen years but knew each other only in a casual way, exchanging "how are you?s" while pulling in and out of our driveways or seeing one another at the occasional party.

But a crisis brought us together on this particular day. Marie had been diagnosed with renal cancer months before and treatment had proved unsuccessful. She had come home to be surrounded by happy memories and by the love and attention of her husband and daughters for whatever time she had left. Paul called that morning because Marie was crying out and in tremendous pain; he had exhausted every method he had been told could help.

I found Marie on a hospital bed in the dining room. The

family had removed all the dining room furniture so that their wife and mother could be in the "center" of the house, wouldn't have to climb stairs, and was near the kitchen and a bathroom. When I spoke to her, Marie was exhausted and tearful, so tormented by this end-stage cancer and its abdominal pain that she could not sleep. Paul ushered me into the kitchen where the counters were overloaded with pill bottles, all of them designed to bring her relief but none of them effective. Turning to me, he said, "Please help us."

Knowing that the family was Catholic, I asked Paul to retrieve a crucifix that hung in their bedroom and we placed it in the dining room over Marie's bed. I explained to Marie that perhaps we could lessen her suffering by teaching her how to elicit the relaxation response. When I explained to her that she needed a word or phrase on which to focus, and that it could be of a religious nature if that would be most soothing to her, she decided upon the rosary. Lying there, taking deep breaths, and holding my hand, Marie focused her mind on a silent iteration of the rosary. Gradually the furrows that accompanied her clenched mouth and eyes smoothed out, and her breathing slowed and became more regular. Within about ten minutes, Marie was asleep. And Paul was relieved, the hours of helplessness at his wife's bedside alleviated at least temporarily.

But a few days later, Paul called me to say that the improvement had been long-lasting and remarkable. Marie was relying primarily on the prayer, refraining from taking almost all the pain medication. Paul related that although Marie was in a great deal of pain, she was free of the terrible distress she had suffered before. And without medication, her mind was clear, her mood brighter. Drawing upon this internal physiologic succor and the power of her beliefs for what turned out to be the final weeks of her life, Marie was at peace when she died.

Another patient of mine, seven years old when I first met him, experienced a liberation of his own by evoking the relaxation response. Andy had been diagnosed with congenital migraine headaches. He had suffered from them since birth, crying almost constantly as a baby. Soon after he could talk, he told his parents that his head hurt.

By the time I saw him, Andy was in the third grade, but he had fallen behind in school and had trouble making friends. In great part this was because Andy often spent full days in darkened rooms, his migraines exacerbated by exposure to bright light. Andy's parents were beside themselves, having pursued the most up-and-coming treatments, but none of the medications or treatments seemed to work.

Andy and his family were also Catholic and we decided on a prayer he could use to activate the relaxation response. Andy made a pact with me to spend ten to twenty minutes silently focused on this prayer twice a day and to use the same approach for a moment or two at the first twinge of a headache. Within a few weeks, Andy could shorten the time the headaches lasted and lengthen the time between headaches. Several weeks later, the severity of the pain decreased. A few months later, Andy's headaches disappeared entirely. His grades and social skills soared, and soon he was playing on the school's hockey team. When I last spoke to the family, Andy was taking no medication and considered the migraines a thing of the past.

Even though Andy and Marie had very different sources of pain, they experienced the same physical event—the relaxation response. No matter what method individuals use to elicit the response, the physiologic changes are the same. The human body is geared to react by providing this calming state—the opposite of the fight-or-flight response—whenever the mind is focused for some time and disregards intrusive, everyday thoughts. In other words, when the mind quiets down, the body follows suit.

So powerful, in fact, is this process that you need not *believe*, you need not call upon remembered wellness to generate the relaxation response. Individuals don't have to say a prayer or anything evocative of their beliefs; they can use any word, phrase, sound, or repetitive activity on which to focus. Just as an injection of penicillin cures strep throat or a laser beam repairs a torn retina, any way you practice the prescribed method of triggering the relaxation response will bring it about, whether or not you believe that it will.

Monkey Mind

T hink of it this way. The fight-or-flight response, your body's reaction to stress, is like that of a fire station responding to a call. All the players need to be dressed in protective gear, equipped, and trained for fire-fighting. Your mind and body make dramatic adjustments for what they believe is an ensuing emergency. Your blood pressure, breathing rate, and speed of metabolism increase; muscle tension also increases and your brain waves become more frequent and intense. On average, you will have a 300 to 400 percent increase of blood flow to the muscles of your arms and legs, all this so that you'll be able to effectively fight or flee.

Most of the stresses we face—probably daily and in some cases many times daily—are false alarms. Yet because the fight-or-flight response is a knee-jerk reaction, ingrained in us as it has been in human physiology for millions of years, we often cannot prevent the mobilization.

Because we do not typically react to a stressful situation with physical exertion, nor do we burn the energy called forth in the fight-or-flight response, we subject ourselves to a legion of negative repercussions. Repeated calls for more forceful propelling of blood throughout the body result in sustained elevations in blood pressure. Higher blood pressure causes enlarged and strained hearts. It also contributes to blockage of arteries—atherosclerosis—and to the bursting of blood vessels, which causes strokes and other forms of internal bleeding. The same adrenaline and noradrenaline can induce cardiac arrhythmias (disturbances in heart rhythms), lower one's threshold for pain, and contribute to higher levels of anxiety, depression, anger, and hostility.

Buddhists have a wonderful term for our churning mental chaos. Literally translated, *papañca* means "monkey mind." Like monkeys jumping from tree limb to tree limb, our minds often leap from thought to thought with little reprieve. When one has a monkey mind, excessive brain activity can overload the system, making it difficult to concentrate, to learn new things, and to fall asleep. Because they are repeatedly instructed to do so, your muscles will also eventually clench out of habit, not just in stressful situations. This muscle tension sends a distress signal to the brain, perpetuating a vicious cycle of physical mobilization for the sake of physical mobilization without relief in sight.

Janet Frank was painfully caught in this vicious cycle when she first came to the Mind/Body Medical Institute two years ago. Mrs. Frank had a severe problem with insomnia; she was lucky if she got to sleep by four or five A.M. even if she'd gone to bed by eleven the night before. Mrs. Frank had never had this problem before. She was, in fact, such a good sleeper that she is the only person I've ever heard of who could actually fall asleep while in the stirrups at her gynecologist's office.

Her sleeping troubles began in 1980 as a result of a very traumatic experience. One day, her eighteen-month-old grandson fell into a swimming pool and nearly drowned, an accident that, tragically, left him both mentally and physically incapacitated. Mrs. Frank spent weeks at a Ronald McDonald House with her son and daughter-in-law, praying and waiting for the little boy to get better. Soon she began experiencing insomnia. "I was bothered by thoughts in my head," she remembers, "about my grandson, and about the difficult relationship I have with my daughter. It was as if their voices were tapes in my head. I couldn't turn them off."

At first, Mrs. Frank just had trouble sleeping in strange places, at friends' homes or in hotels; gradually she stopped going places for fear of being unable to sleep. Unfortunately, the problem worsened. Eventually she couldn't sleep even in her own house, so Mrs. Frank stayed up all night, listening to talk radio, making muffins, catching up on ironing, and walking around the house for hours at a time. Since her husband had died years before and her children were grown and out of the house, she didn't have to worry about disturbing anyone. But the problem was maddening and the fatigue made her very susceptible to illness.

She had checked *The Relaxation Response* out of the library and had tried practicing meditation on her own. But when she read in an insurance newsletter that treatment for insomnia at the Mind/Body Medical Institute was covered, she came in to see Dr. Gregg D. Jacobs, my colleague who specializes in insomnia treatment.

Before she began eliciting the relaxation response, Mrs. Frank always needed the radio on to go to sleep, because the voices it broadcast overcame the voices in her head. But when she lay down and recited "The Lord is my shepherd" or "Give me peace" to herself, her heart stopped beating as hard as it used to and she could drop off to sleep. She explains, "I would visualize God and I could almost see God watching over me. God would calm me down. I could almost reach out and touch him, that's how real it was to me."

Mrs. Frank called upon the power of the top-down capacity of her brain to make her belief real to her. Then, she applied her belief to a mental focusing mechanism that brings forth the physical relaxation she described. Fortunately, not only are our hearts wired to pump rapidly when we're under stress, they're also wired for the opposite effect, for a balm that can counteract the damaging consequences of stress.

The relaxation response isn't as quickly mobilized as the fight-or-flight response, which is needed in emergencies. Nor does it, in modern life, usually come without being called, although many of us have probably triggered the relaxation response in our bodies without knowing it. Our ancestors unwittingly evoked the relaxation response even more frequently because they so often gazed at sunsets or stared at the horizon. They did not have Nintendo or video rentals to entertain and distract them, nor a popular culture that aspired to keep them perpetually excited and aroused. But even if it was more common for our ancestors to enjoy quiet and uninterrupted solace, we maintain the ability to elicit and reap the same rewards they did from the relaxation response.

When you focus for a short time, gently brushing aside any intrusive thoughts, your mind and body suddenly become a five-star resort in which all the service personnel make your restoration and health their priority and are especially concerned with alleviating the harmful effects of stress. This great

TABLE 2

COMPARISON OF THE PHYSIOLOGIC CHANGES OF THE FIGHT-OR-FLIGHT RESPONSE AND THE RELAXATION RESPONSE

PHYSIOLOGIC STATE	FIGHT-OR-FLIGHT RESPONSE	RELAXATION RESPONSE
Metabolism	Increases	Decreases
Blood Pressure	Increases	Decreases
Heart Rate	Increases	Decreases
Rate of Breathing	Increases	Decreases
Blood Flowing to the Muscles of the Arms and Legs	Increases	Stable
Muscle Tension	Increases	Decreases
Slow Brain Waves	Decrease	Increase

team of stress-busters and body-relaxers emerges when everyday thoughts and worries are put aside. The table above shows the stark contrast in bodily changes brought on by the activation of the fight-or-flight response as compared to that of the relaxation response (see Table 2).

Characteristics of the Relaxation Response

A hallmark feature of the relaxation response is a significant decrease in the body's oxygen consumption, or hypometabolism. The cells in your body use oxygen from the air you breathe to burn the nutrients from the food you eat. This is metabolism, or the process by which the body burns or consumes oxygen and uses generated energy to permit your brain, heart, lungs, and other parts of your body to function properly. The body responds to techniques that elicit the relaxation response by downshifting your metabolism, by allowing your internal perpetual-energy machine to ease off working so hard. Much less fuel is needed to sustain the body in the hypometabolic state characteristic of the relaxation response. Your heart need not beat so quickly, your blood need not be pumped as forcefully. Your breathing can be slower and deeper, and your muscles relaxed and requiring less blood. The ever-vigilant and active organs of your body, which are often forced to spring into maximum speed and production at a hint of trouble, can relish for a few moments a less demanding schedule of outputs and requirements. It's like giving a hyperenergetic kindergartner an afternoon nap.

This reaction is exactly opposite to the fight-or-flight response in which the body upshifts from its average, at-rest metabolic rate into hypermetabolism. When the brain gets a signal to change, adjust, or react to a threat—coming from the body or the environment in bottom-up messages or from a thought or perception in top-down signals—oxygen consumption and metabolism accelerate to produce more fuel for the body so it can fight or flee.

The body does shift into a hypometabolic state when we sleep. And incidentally, animals experience hypometabolism both during sleep and hibernation—facts that first led me to consider that perhaps the relaxation response could be a previously unrecognized human capacity for hibernation. But one of the defining characteristics of hibernation found in animals, the decrease in body temperature, was not true of those eliciting the relaxation response.

As far as science knows, the calming effects of the relaxation response cannot be brought about as dramatically or as quickly by any other means. Sure, the body's metabolism slows down when you lie in a hammock, watch TV, or read a book. But it does not slow to the significant degree that it does in the relaxation response or sleep. And oxygen consumption decreases much faster in the relaxation response than in sleep. When you shut off the light and sink into your pillow at night, your oxygen consumption very gradually decreases until four or five hours later, when it levels out at an average of 8 percent less than the rate you experience when you're awake and at rest. When instructions to elicit the relaxation response are followed, however, the decrease is dramatic and immediate, on average decreasing by 10 to 17 percent within the first three minutes.

Although we still need to learn more about how slower waves experienced in the relaxation response affect the brain and our moods, we know that higher frequency beta rhythms dominate the brain during the majority of our wakeful hours, when we are engaged in everyday thinking and under stress. Slower brain waves summoned in the relaxation response are often linked to feelings of pleasure. It appears that drawing upon different brain rhythms and patterns enhances both our moods and our health.

The Long-Term Effects

Regular elicitation of the relaxation response is of enormous benefit to your body. Tuning out everyday worries, breaking that mental tumult known as monkey mind, you give the body permission to relax. And just as repeated activation of the fight-or-flight response can lead to sustained problems in the body and its mechanics, so too can repeated activation of the relaxation response reverse those trends and mend the internal wear and tear brought on by stress.

Our bodies are engaged in a kind of tug-of-war, stress on one end of the rope and relaxation on the other. But given the amount of tension we experience every day, the quick pace and the enormous expectations we have of ourselves in modern times and particularly in urban life, the teams have never seemed very fair, stress always seeming to overcome relaxation. But regular elicitation of the relaxation response evens the teams, the cumulative effects of relaxation countering the cumulative effects of stress, making a healthy equilibrium possible.

How to Elicit the Relaxation Response

T he steps to evoking the relaxation response are not necessarily difficult or unusual. To enjoy the relaxation response, both its short-term calming effects and its long-term contribution to health, choose a technique that conforms to your own beliefs. The relaxation response can be evoked by any of a large number of techniques, including meditation, certain types of prayer, autogenic training, progressive muscular relaxation, jogging, swimming, Lamaze breathing exercises, yoga, tai chi chuan, chi gong, and even knitting and crocheting.

Only two basic steps need to be followed. You need to repeat a word, sound, prayer, phrase, or muscular activity. And when common, everyday thoughts intrude on your focus, passively disregard them and return to your repetition (see Table 3).

The choice of a focused repetition is up to the individual. You can choose any focus, but to enhance the benefits of the relaxation response with the effects of remembered wellness and to ensure that you will adhere to the routine of eliciting it, the focus should be appropriate. If you are a religious person, you can choose a prayer; if you are a nonreligious person, choose a secular focus. The relaxation response and remembered wellness are a very potent pair, the combined force of which we will discuss in the next chapter. Regardless of the technique or focus you select, the relaxation response will be evoked if you use the two steps—the repetition of a focus and the passive disregard of interfering thoughts with a return to the focus.

TABLE 3
THE TWO STEPS
TO ELICITING THE RELAXATION RESPONSE

1. Repeat a word, sound, prayer, phrase, or muscular activity.
2. Passively disregard everyday thoughts that come to mind, and return to your repetition.

TABLE 4
SECULAR FOCUS WORDS

One	Ocean	Love	Peace	Calm	Relax

There is no "Benson technique" for eliciting the relaxation response. In fact, my colleagues and I offer people a smorgasbord of techniques and focuses. Sometimes patients tell me they like having an instructor decide on a focus or assign one to them. Evidently, for these people, it lends more credence or meaning to the focus for them if a doctor, nurse, clergyperson, or another leader helps them choose it. Again, this is a product of remembered wellness: The trust you place in a caregiver adds power to the process. The point is, any focus will work, and if you like the sound of one that is given to you, try it.

Here are some very common focus words, phrases, and prayers that may help you get started (see Tables 4 and 5).

While adherence to the two steps—repetition and passive

TABLE 5
RELIGIOUS FOCUS WORDS OR PRAYERS

Christian (Protestant or Catholic)
   "Our Father who art in heaven"
   "The Lord is my shepherd"

Catholic
   "Hail, Mary, full of grace"
   "Lord Jesus Christ, have mercy on me"

Jewish
   "Sh'ma Yisroel"
   "Shalom"
   "Echod"
   "The Lord is my shepherd"

Islamic
   "Insha'allah"

Hindu
   "Om"

disregard for intrusive thoughts—readily evokes the relaxation response no matter how and where they're performed, the following is the generic technique I teach to patients and which I have used myself for many years:

Step 1. Pick a focus word or short phrase that's firmly rooted in your belief system.

Step 2. Sit quietly in a comfortable position.

Step 3. Close your eyes.

Step 4. Relax your muscles.

Step 5. Breathe slowly and naturally, and as you do, repeat your focus word, phrase, or prayer silently to yourself as you exhale.

Step 6. Assume a passive attitude. Don't worry about how well you're doing. When other thoughts come to mind, simply say to yourself, "Oh, well," and gently return to the repetition.

Step 7. Continue for ten to twenty minutes.

Step 8. Do not stand immediately. Continue sitting quietly for a minute or so, allowing other thoughts to return. Then open your eyes and sit for another minute before rising.

Step 9. Practice this technique once or twice daily.

In this generic technique, I suggest that you sit quietly in a comfortable position, close your eyes, and relax your muscles. However, you can also do it with your eyes open; you can kneel, you can stand and sway, or you can adopt the lotus position so many people associate with meditation.

You can also jog and elicit the relaxation response, paying attention to the cadence of your feet on the pavement—"left, right, left, right"—and when other thoughts come into your head, say, "Oh, well," and return to "left, right, left, right." Of course you must keep your eyes open! We have found that by using this approach, the runner will achieve in the first mile the "runner's high" that usually occurs in the third or fourth mile.

Several years ago I was addressing a luncheon of armed service chaplains in Texas and met an army general, the highest ranking clergyman in the United States. This Catholic priest told me that he had always tried to be efficient by saying his prayers and exercising at the same time. When he jogged, he had always repeated to himself the Jesus prayer—"Lord Jesus, have mercy on me." But unbeknownst to him until that meeting, he had achieved even more efficiency—exercising, praying, and eliciting the relaxation response all at once!

The Focused Walk

My friend T George Harris, editor-in-chief of both *Psychology Today* and *American Health*, as well as the editor of the *Harvard Business Review*, has collaborated with writer Linus Mundy to produce *Prayer Walking*, a small guide that offers many great insights for those "on the path to body-and-soul fitness." Available through Abbey Press, this tiny volume speaks volumes about the benefits of "taking a trip"—not a vacation, but simply a short break in which we walk away from our everyday environments where our brains are bustling and our bodies exhausting themselves rising to meet stressful occasions.

Our research has shown that performing a focused exercise activates the relaxation response. In 1978, we found that when you exercise and simultaneously focus your mind, your exercise becomes more efficient—that is, you require less energy to do physical work. Furthermore, in research that the generous support of my friends Ruth Strickler and her husband, Bruce Dayton, made possible, Dr. Youde Wang and other colleagues at the University of Massachusetts found that focused walking was associated with reduced anxiety and diminished negative thoughts. Similar results were achieved during a mindful exercise, a version of tai chi chuan developed by Ms. Strickler at her health club, The Marsh, in Minnetonka, Minnesota. No such positive mood changes were found to be present in unfocused walking.

So instead of the radio station you usually tune into on your Walkman, try tuning down the noise of the world to which you are so accustomed. By exercising and eliciting the response, you cover many of the bases to promote good health.

Sitting or standing, walking or swimming, even knitting and crocheting. it is the repetitive quality of the exercise that helps engender the relaxation response. In the same way that a parent can be assured of a few moments of rest by putting a baby in an automatic swing, the brain and the body can take advantage of the rest inherent in an easy, repetitive task, creating a kind of hypnotic effect. There are two stages to hypnosis: the presuggestion stage, and the suggestion phase in which a person, for example, could be instructed to "levitate" or raise an arm. The presuggestion phase is the same physiologic state as the relaxation response. And as in hypnosis, people eliciting the relaxation response open a kind of door, clearing and rejuvenating their minds and bodies, readying themselves for new ideas and suggestions.

Silencing the Chaos Within

I believe the shift in brain waves I mentioned earlier is, in part, responsible for the "door-opening effect" that so many people experience as a result of eliciting the relaxation response. People emerge from mental focusing with clearer minds and sharper thoughts. The brain seems to use the quiet time to wipe the slate clean so that new ideas and beliefs can present themselves. Many of us try to keep the brain as busy and active as possible, but I've learned that a period of brain focusing to the exclusion of everyday thoughts can actually increase mental productivity.

The affirmations and visualizations I mentioned earlier are particularly helpful when used right after eliciting the response. It appears that the mind is more receptive and that you can restructure what may be a pattern of negative thinking with these exercises. This is cognitive restructuring in which thoughts are redirected to interpret life events in a more positive, more realistic fashion. As damaging as negativity is (and this book has revealed much of this), we need strategies to reprogram the soft and changeable wirings of the brain in order to remember wellness.

A former patient of mine and now a colleague who teaches mental focusing in his classroom, Ron Banister, will attest to this fact. Mr. Banister is a musician and jazz instructor at the New England Conservatory of Music in Boston. He elicits the relaxation response to silence the chaos within.

Mr. Banister does not use a prayer or scripture, nor does he call upon God or a religious belief. He invokes "art" to generate the response, often using the name of the great jazz pianist Thelonious Monk as his focus or mantra. This is but one step in his three-step process to enhance his health and professional ability. The second is a "focused listening" exercise in which he centers his attention on random sounds or on certain passages of music, and the third taking in a host of what he calls "vitamins"—songs from favorite artists such as Ray Charles and Billie Holiday that revive him.

"Ear training" is an important component of musical training, central to both Mr. Banister's own performance and to his teaching. Mr. Banister teaches young musicians to recognize different hues in music, paying close attention to "violence" in music in gangster films or the dark accompaniments in film noir, and developing long-term memory for various movements of orchestras or jazz ensembles. Eliciting the relaxation response sharpens the musician's ear, he thinks, by giving the mind "a concrete focus" and dismissing extraneous thoughts and sounds.

Mr. Banister says that not only does the elicitation liberate his mind, it lubricates it, as if unleashing a muse. Often afterward, Mr. Banister will sit down at the piano and improvise, letting his subconscious emerge on the keys, allowing himself what he calls "full colors" without worrying about producing music. Sometimes, he says, the results are surprising and interesting; other times they are less remarkable. Nevertheless, this "shuttle between the abstract and concrete" feels very healthy, both for him and his music.

In his book *The Man Who Tasted Shapes*, neurologist Dr. Cytowic describes his first experience with a form of Buddhist meditation. Clark, a trusted friend, had encouraged him to sit in front of a blank wall with his eyes open, instructing him,

"Neither try to think nor try not to think. When the opposites arise the Buddha mind is lost. Just sitting with no deliberate thought is the important part of Zazen," the type of meditation they were trying to achieve. A neurologist, Dr. Cytowic protested that he did not believe that it was physically possible "for 'nothing' to be going on in one's mind." But Clark egged him on, saying, "This isn't something that you question because it doesn't have a rational answer. It's just something that you do."

So Dr. Cytowic did it. He concentrated on the blank wall until he touched what he calls "the still point." And he writes, "My cognitive mind was astonished that the internal dialogue really could be stopped, while the rest of me relished the sense of tranquillity that accompanied this feat. It is a feeling [that] must be experienced to be understood, because it cannot be explained."

I like Dr. Cytowic's account of his first experience with meditation precisely because he explains a seemingly unexplainable experience so well, and because his friend Clark told him what I so often have to tell my patients about the task of focusing the mind. I encourage people to make the elicitation of the relaxation response part of their daily routine, but not to aspire to good results or some specific end. "Just do it," as the slogan goes.

Like Brushing Your Teeth

Try to think of the practice as you would the daily ritual of brushing your teeth, which all of us were taught to do before we even got a permanent set. Because this habit was formed so long ago, when we were children—perhaps our parents even withheld bedtime stories until the deed was done—it's a "no-brainer." We do it naturally, sometimes even when we're half-awake. But when we're finished, we don't grade the experience, thinking that was a "good brush" or "bad brush."

Let your body heal itself without the interference of mind-generated doubts, criticism, and appraisals. (Doubts, criticism, and judgments, of course, register a threat in your mind, arousing the mind and body and initiating the fight-or-flight response.) You wouldn't critique your toothbrushing so don't analyze this exercise either. Let the ten to twenty minutes you plan into your schedule twice each day become a no-brainer, a break from the usual harried thinking with which you conscientiously approach other activities in your life.

I know this is hard for many of my patients because people who are concerned enough about their health and well-being to learn relaxation response techniques are usually very motivated and disciplined. Just as science and a science-minded society has trained them to do, they look for measurable results. When the ten to twenty minutes is up, they want to take their pulse and report a decreased heart rate, and almost certainly their heart rate will be slower.

But you won't elicit the relaxation response when your concentration is interrupted by thoughts such as "How am I doing?," "Is it working?," "Did I achieve the goal?" You won't achieve a goal of calmness by checking on your progress because inevitably, even though it's only subconscious, you'll be too engaged in arousing thoughts to fully center your attention on the focus that brings the relaxation response about in the first place.

The relaxation response works because it breaks the train of everyday thought. It gives the brain and thus the body a respite because, for a few minutes, the mechanisms required for us to think, act, move, chew, or smell are taken off the full-alert mode in which we usually function. If you don't let go of the full-alert mode, you won't garner the rewards.

Let Go of Worry

As members of a society fixated on self-help, most of us are accustomed to doctors, dietitians, exercise physiologists, and other advisers telling us to journal or chart our progress. We expect results, if not right away on the bathroom scale, then at least in a few weeks when bathing suit season arrives. We are used to competing, if not with others, at least with ourselves.

My writing collaborator Marg Stark remembers her first yoga classes in which she had to adapt to an exercise that didn't involve competition. Yoga was entirely different from aerobic classes in which Marg always felt pressure to keep up with the instructor and other class members, even if she was a beginner, even if she could barely walk to her car after pushing herself too hard through the first class. In yoga, Marg learned that longtime yoga practitioners could "go deeper," benefiting from the same simple exercises and stretches taught to beginners. Moreover, yoga attracted men and women of all ages, and the goal was not to look good in Spandex but to relax, increase flexibility, relieve pain, and gain strength. Yoga was, in fact, unlike any sport or athletic endeavor Marg had ever experienced, so free of competition and self-consciousness that she no longer had to battle her own sense of pride to do something good for herself.

Yoga and all the other methods of eliciting the relaxation response have this in common: The less you worry about the results, the better. Just let it happen. Again, this advice tends to be hard to swallow in a society that, to a certain extent, prizes worry because it motivates us, because it causes a rush of adrenaline that makes us perform better. But the truth is, most of us worry far too much about far too many things instead of reserving worry and the body-alerting effect of the fight-or-flight response for crucial matters.

I encourage my patients to direct their worry about their bodies and the discipline that led them to pursue treatment into a disciplined practice of relaxation response techniques. Use that initial worry to make sure you adhere to the routine. Just experience the calming effects and let me quantify the results at your checkups, I tell them.

Do It Just for the Sake of Doing It

This is a good skill to learn, eliciting the relaxation response for the sake of doing it, not because you have been conditioned to believe that you must meet some goal or report some results. It's no different from what we already instinctively know—that taking a walk after a stressful day is good for us. In general, we don't have to dissect or assign specific values to this "stuff of life." Quite ironically, when we do, we undermine not only our enjoyment and experience of life but the specific and measurable benefits that science is now telling us can be culled from such activities.

One other misconception can stand in the way of enjoying the benefits of the relaxation response. Many people have heard and been conditioned to expect that meditation and prayer bring "altered consciousness," or that they can result in "peak" spiritual or mystical enlightenment. So if the relaxation response isn't mind-blowing in proportion, we think it isn't working or that it's not doing anything. Again, I encourage my patients not to expect fireworks, just to perform the steps without a great deal of reflection or anticipation.

You'll remember that Mrs. Frank used a visualization during her elicitation of the relaxation response, trying to picture the Lord she was invoking in her prayer. Visualizations are very powerful mind exercises, as I explained in the section on top-down-generated thoughts. Visualizations send signals to the brain that arise not from the body itself, not from the environment, but from your imagination or memories. Similarly, many people enjoy using affirmations after eliciting the relaxation response, when the mind is open and ready for new concepts. Physiologically, this is the perfect time to introduce positive messages, to restructure your thoughts, and to rid your mind of the destructive thinking that can engage the nocebo effect.

Once people make the elicitation part of their daily routine, I also encourage them to use "minis." Minis are bite-size versions of the relaxation response, the simple act of breath-

ing deeply, releasing physical tension, and saying your chosen
focus word, sound, prayer, or phrase to yourself on your outbreaths when you feel stress getting the best of you in the
midst of your day.

Cumulative Effects

At the Mind/Body Medical Institute, we recommend
that the elicitation of the relaxation response be
combined with other self-care techniques such as nutrition, exercise, and stress management. This complete program is described in a book my colleague Eileen M. Stewart
RN, C, MS, other members of the Mind/Body Medical Institute, and I have compiled entitled *The Wellness Book.* Most
people feel some effects of these lifestyle changes immediately, but the larger, more dramatic effects of the relaxation
response are cumulative. In the tug-of-war I alluded to earlier,
the mind/body needs time to even the teams, countering the
fight-or-flight with the relaxation response over an extended
period in which an individual elicits the response daily.

When I met him in 1986, Jimmy Burke had already endured two years of one long anxiety attack. At first, maybe two
or three times a year, he experienced the classic symptoms of
an anxiety attack—dizziness, headaches, tightness in his chest,
breathing difficulties, sometimes even hyperventilating—for
about five minutes. But one morning, he woke up and felt an
intense fright. It gripped him very hard and did not go away
after a few minutes, a few hours, a few days and even months
later. A plumber, Mr. Burke barely got through his work every
day, and felt like he was "living on the edge." He took tranquilizers, he went to therapy, he saw several specialists in
Boston but couldn't get any relief. Eventually he began drinking very heavily, leaning on alcohol to calm him in whatever
way it could.

"I was searching for anything," Mr. Burke remembers. "I was
desperate." Someone at work asked him if he'd tried meditation
and gave him my name. When Mr. Burke came to see me, I laid

out the progress he could expect to see as a result of the elicitation, based on the experiences other patients had had.

He recalls, "Dr. Benson told me that within six months,
we'd try to cut back to one-third of the medications I had
been taking, and that after a year, I'd be medication-free. I
wanted to believe him so badly. He was the only doctor who
seemed sure that he could help me."

Mr. Burke took part in a program at the Mind/Body Medical Institute in which he was introduced to about twenty
other people, all of them experiencing different medical
problems. He remembers that in addition to the relaxation
response, he learned about self-esteem and positive thinking.
In the beginning, he came to see me once a week.

Within a few months of his first visit, the anxiety attack Mr.
Burke had endured for two years began to subside. He says
that sometimes, after a hard day, he'll take time out for a mini
and he'll feel so energized that it's as if he's napped for three
hours. Today, nearly ten years later, he has to laugh when people tell him how "laid-back" he seems. And Mr. Burke says he
is "95 percent cured," remembering that I told him it could
take ten years to counter and reverse the incredible influence
stress had had on his body.

"To think that I sat in front of a therapist for months and
months!" he exclaims. "We never found out what brought it
on. It's the same as when you get an ulcer. Nobody knows
what exactly brings this on. It's just things in your life . . . I was
in Dr. Benson's waiting room one time and another trades-
man was there with the same symptoms I had had. He told me
that he just couldn't find the time for the focusing exercise,
and I said, 'You haven't got the time not to do it!' "

Life Changes

Many of my patients report a lifestyle change, a calm
that extends long after the elicitation is finished. My
colleague John Hoffman, Ph.D., and I found that after exposure to the relaxation response, the body requires

more of the hormone noradrenaline to increase heart rate and blood pressure—a blocking effect previously only partly achieved with the use of several categories of drugs, the so-called alpha- and beta-blockers. Moreover, these drugs cause side effects and do not produce the other positive changes brought on by the relaxation response. The relaxation response nullifies, to a certain extent, the action of noradrenaline, so that the body does not react as radically to mildly stressful events but retains the ability to respond immediately to major threats. In this way, people with hypertension can experience long-term relief with the relaxation response.

For all patients, the relaxation response is not only a short-term boon but a long-term balm. My colleagues and I at the Mind/Body Medical Institute have amassed evidence of the tremendous diversity of medical conditions that the elicitation, together with other self-care strategies such as nutrition, exercise, and stress-management, can heal or cure (principal investigators are listed after each study; Dr. Richard Friedman, research director of the Mind/Body Medical Institute, made major contributions to most of these research projects):

- Patients with hypertension experienced significant decreases in blood pressure and needed fewer or no medications over a three-year measurement period (Eileen M. Stewart, RN, C, MS).
- Patients with chronic pain experienced less severity of pain, more activity, less anxiety, less depression, less anger, and they visited the managed care facility where they received care 36 percent less often in the two years after completing the program than they did prior to treatment (Margaret A. Caudill, MD, Ph.D.).
- Seventy-five percent of patients with sleep-onset insomnia (meaning that they couldn't fall asleep easily) were cured and became normal sleepers. Sleeping also improved for the other 25 percent, and most patients took significantly fewer sleep medications (Gregg D. Jacobs, Ph.D.).

- Thirty-six percent of women with unexplained infertility became pregnant within six months of completing the program (Alice D. Domar, Ph.D.).
- Patients with complaints described by the admitting personnel as psychosomatic and who were frequent users of a health maintenance organization reduced their number of visits by 50 percent (Caroline J.C. Hellman, Ph.D.).
- Women suffering from symptoms of premenstrual syndrome (PMS) experienced a 57 percent decrease in severity. The more severe the PMS, the more effective the relief with the relaxation response (Irene L. Goodale, Ph.D.).
- Patients with cancer and AIDS experienced decreased symptoms and better control of nausea and vomiting associated with chemotherapy (Ann Webster, Ph.D.).
- Patients with cardiac arrhythmias experienced fewer of them (Herbert Benson, MD).
- Patients who suffered from anxiety or mild or moderate depression were less anxious, depressed, angry, and hostile (Herbert Benson, MD).
- Patients undergoing painful X-ray procedures experienced less anxiety and pain and needed one-third the amount of pain and anxiety medications usually required (Carol L. Mandle, RN, Ph.D.).
- Patients who had open-heart surgery had fewer postoperative arrhythmias and less anxiety following surgery (Jane Lesserman, Ph.D.).
- Migraine and cluster headache sufferers found they had fewer and less severe headaches (Herbert Benson, MD).
- High school sophomores increased their self-esteem (Herbert Benson, MD).
- Working people experienced reduced symptoms of depression, anxiety, and hostility (Patricia Carrington, Ph.D.).
- Working people had fewer medical symptoms,

fewer illness days, improved performance, and
lower blood pressure (Ruanne K. Peters, SD).

To the extent that any condition is caused or worsened by
stress, the relaxation response or relaxation-response-based
programs practiced at the Deaconess Hospital can be effective
at curing or improving the condition. This is extremely important, since 60 to 90 percent of all doctor office visits in this
country are stress-related and fall within the realm of maladies
that mind/body medicine can alleviate. These conditions are
poorly treated by two of the legs in the three-legged stool,
namely medications and surgical procedures.

Although it's clear that all of us have the ability to evoke its
great effects, we still don't precisely know which brain mechanisms make the relaxation response possible. And while the
relaxation response has stood up to distinctions science has
demanded and proved itself separate from remembered wellness, these distinctions feel unnatural to patients, as we'll explore in the next chapter. Readily mingled, it is as if we are
wired to experience the two of them in combination. And so
my search continued.

CHAPTER 7

THE FAITH FACTOR AND THE SPIRITUAL EXPERIENCE

You saw in the previous chapter how I suggested to patients that they pick pleasing or soothing words or phrases on which to focus their minds in order to elicit the relaxation response. You also read that patients have often chosen to focus on words or phrases that are religious or spiritual in nature. Although I wanted patients to enjoy the technique so that they would adhere to its practice, and I wanted them to reap the rewards of remembered wellness by believing in the technique, the tendency of most to choose prayer as a focus was surprising to me. Because as I tried to emphasize the physiologic benefits of the relaxation response, my patients impressed upon me the spiritual qualities of the experience, leading my scientific projects into the nonscientific realm of religion.

In this chapter, I'll continue to demonstrate how patients naturally combined the relaxation response and remembered wellness. But it wasn't just belief in themselves or belief in the technique that they applied to mental focusing, it was often religious faith. That's why I came to call the combination of these physiologic powers "the faith factor" (I'll give the full definition in a moment). As you will begin to glimpse in this chapter, my identification of the faith factor had tremendous repercussions. More and more, I was drawn toward something physically lasting and true about human beings. But simultaneously, I was coming closer to defining a biological role of belief in God, a line of inquiry that I wasn't sure either scientists or theologians would appreciate.

A Physician Teaching Prayer

Several years ago, T George Harris, who you'll recall from the last chapter served as editor for several magazines, introduced me to venture capitalist and philanthropist Laurance S. Rockefeller. Harris told me that Mr. Rockefeller was a deeply spiritual person who would undoubtedly be interested in my findings, and accordingly, I was invited to dinner at Pocantico, the Rockefeller complex in the Hudson River Valley in New York state, where I told Mr. Rockefeller about my work. More specifically, I told him that 80 percent of my patients picked prayers as the focus of their elicitation, be they Jewish, Christian, Buddhist, or Hindu. Because the vast majority of patients chose to enrich the medical therapy with their faith, I often found myself in a peculiar position—that of a physician teaching people to pray.

Mr. Rockefeller was very interested in this, and he went on to demonstrate his interest by underwriting some conferences on the subject (I'll talk about this later in this chapter). I also described to him the research I did that led up to the unintended consequences of my becoming a physician who taught people to pray. Because not only did 80 percent of my patients choose a religious focus for their elicitation, but about 25 percent of my patients reported feeling "more spiritual" as a result of eliciting the relaxation response, whether they chose a religious or a secular focus. And our 25 percent rate may be conservative considering that a 1994 *Newsweek* poll revealed that 45 percent of people polled had "sensed the sacred" during meditation.

A Spiritual Tendency

In some respects, this propensity for "spirituality" reminds me of the tendency of people to describe near-death experiences as spiritual. Medicine can, to a certain extent, explain the physical processes that cause people on the brink of dying to "see light" and experience joy and peace—a lack of oxygen to the brain causes the cells involved in their vision to register tunnels of light, and a release of endorphins causes the pleasurable sensations. Nevertheless, people are convinced that these near-death experiences are religious.

Trends like these intrigued me, because everything I'd learned about remembered wellness taught me that beliefs of all kinds could be influential in health. And once again, the dichotomies between mind and matter, between science and religion, seemed to be going against the grain of people's natural reactions and, especially important to me, against the interactions of verifiable, physiologic assets—namely, remembered wellness and the relaxation response.

I began to ask myself, why are spiritual or mystical experiences some of the most desired and sought after of life experiences? I had had some strange events happen in my life that could be considered prophetic. For instance, my mother claims that, as a toddler, one of the first words I uttered was "doctor." So improbable is this that I used to suspect that it came as the result of considerable coaching. Other times I thought that Mom revised history to make my choice of a profession seem ordained. But she always stood by her story, so over the years I've accepted her version of my "calling" to medicine.

I went on to have other extremely fortuitous and improbable encounters. One incident occurred when I was sixteen, the morning after I had camped out on Jones Beach on Long Island with my friend Howard Rotner. By modern standards, this must seem unusual in and of itself—that a beach a half hour outside New York City was considered so harmless that our parents let us spend the night there. But in those days the beach was open and perfectly safe, even for unaccompanied teenagers, and we liked nothing more than these overnight summer adventures.

Early in the morning, having stayed up all night on a damp, isolated stretch of sand, I was playing with a string of kelp on the beach, tearing it apart to see what was inside. I was approached by an elderly woman who was wearing an ankle-length cotton dress and a black macramé shawl and was hunched over a cane. She seemed to have stepped right out of an illustrated fairy tale, so perfectly cast was she for a fortune-telling role. This stranger came up to me and said, "You're going to be a doctor someday," and without another word, proceeded down the beach, eventually disappearing from view. To my knowledge, I had never seen this woman before nor did I ever see her again. (Incidentally, Howard Rotner went on to become a physician as well.)

I found myself the subject of yet another unlikely happenstance during my first year of medical school. I was out on a date with a woman who had spent much of our time together disparaging the field of medicine, so unenthused was she with my choice of career. We sat down on the lawn by a small river near the Harvard Medical School campus where we had been walking when out of nowhere a bird dropped from the sky and fell on the grass right beside us. The bird, a starling, was still alive, thrashing and chirping, trying to fly away but only managing to jump a few inches. Gently, I scooped the bird up and, acting on instinct, I pulled and reset what appeared to be a dislocated wing, placed the bird on the grass, and watched as it fluttered and flew quickly away. I was astounded. But my date was flabbergasted, and gracious enough to retract what she had said just minutes before about the limited merits of my "calling."

Spiritual Experiences

At one time or another, I'm sure nearly everyone experiences extraordinary and magical events such as this, the converging of time and circumstance so logic-defiant that one cannot help but feel these events were divinely directed. It could be a chance reunion with a long-lost friend, a life change that comes at precisely the time you need it, or an image you see in a cloud formation. It could be a clergyperson's sermon that seems eerily relevant to the problems you've been facing, something as dramatic as hearing a voice speak to you inspirationally or as quiet as a bliss that envelops you suddenly. Whatever the form, the more the incident means to us, the more we attach sacred status to it in our lives. We shake our heads, asking, "What are the chances?," all the while feeling a profound reverberation within that perhaps life is not random, that perhaps these are tangible signs that a mystical force contours our life experiences.

But it's possible that the reverberation you feel within, when an experience you deem magical or spiritual occurs, may not just be emotional but physical as well. Not only did my research—and that of my colleagues—reveal that 25 percent of people feel more spiritual as the result of the elicitation of the relaxation response, but it showed that those same people have fewer medical symptoms than do those who reported no increase in spirituality from the elicitation.

The Faith Factor

I decided to call the combined force of these internal influences the faith factor—remembered wellness and the elicitation of the relaxation response. But it became clear that a person's religious convictions or life philosophy enhanced the average effects of the relaxation response in three ways: 1) People who chose an appropriate focus, that which draws upon their deepest philosophic or religious convictions, were more apt to adhere to the elicitation routine, looking forward to it and enjoying it; 2) Affirmative beliefs of any kind brought forth remembered wellness, reviving top-down, nerve-cell-firing patterns in the brain that were associated with wellness; 3) When present, faith in an eternal or life-transcending force seemed to make the fullest use of remembered wellness because it is a supremely soothing belief, disconnecting unhealthy logic and worries.

I already knew that eliciting the relaxation response could "disconnect" everyday thoughts and worries, calming people's bodies and minds more quickly and to a degree otherwise unachievable. It appeared that beliefs added to the response transported the mind/body even more dramatically, quieting worries and fears significantly better than the relaxation response alone. And I speculated that religious faith was more influential than other affirmative beliefs.

At her early age, Anne Frank wrote in the diary that she kept while hiding from would-be Nazi captors, "He who has courage and faith will never perish in misery." I began to believe that she was right, that a belief in God dispatched by our brains is deeply soothing to our bodies.

I want to emphasize that the benefits of the faith factor are not the exclusive domain of the devout. People don't have to have a professed belief in God to reap the psychological and physical rewards of the faith factor. With lead investigator Dr. Jared D. Kass, a professor at Lesley College Graduate School of Arts and Sciences in Cambridge, Massachusetts, my colleagues and I developed a questionnaire to quantify and describe the spiritual feelings that accompanied the relaxation response, to document their frequency as well as their potential health effects.

Based on the survey responses, we calculated "spirituality scores." But because virtually all of our survey respondents reported a "belief in God," this statement could not be used to differentiate people. It was the more amorphous feeling of spirituality that could be linked to better psychological and physical well-being. However, there is one group that does seem more likely to have spiritual encounters. Indeed, women had higher spirituality scores than men, for reasons we don't yet understand.

Immediate and Cumulative Effects

Our studies demonstrated that people feel an increase in spirituality relatively quickly upon eliciting the relaxation response but that the longer one makes the elicitation part of one's routine, the more these sensations grow. Like the physical rewards we had measured, spirituality also seemed to be cumulative, increasing over time as people regularly elicited the response.

Again under Dr. Kass's leadership, our research group found that those who elicited the relaxation response regularly for more than one month had higher spirituality scores than those who did so less than one month. It didn't matter if you were a novice or an old-timer, religious or nonreligious; the effects and rewards of the faith factor proved possible for very diverse individuals.

But what exactly were people experiencing that felt spiritual to them? When we compiled the results, some common themes emerged. People who reported increased spirituality after eliciting the relaxation response described two things about the experience: 1) the presence of an energy, a force, a power—God—that was beyond themselves, and 2) this presence felt close to them. And it was the people who "felt this presence" who noted the greatest medical benefits. Regardless of their professed faith, people eliciting the response who experienced these sensations—an energy that seemed both internal and external to their bodies, and that felt good—had better health as a result.

The Energy Force

Many people ask me if I attribute this perceived force to "chi," the energy that traditional Chinese and other Eastern medical practitioners believe pulses through us and through the natural world. Western scientists do not acknowledge these energies, although some would agree that there is a life force, a spirit, or a soul that breathes life into bodies. But many cultures have named and believed in a mysterious healing energy. The ancient Egyptians called it "Ka," the Hawaiians "Mana," and the Indians "Prana." In these cultures, people believe that healers can direct and restore these healing forces.

Using standard scientific methods, I have tried to isolate and measure chi, or this energy to which so many cultures ascribe medicinal benefits, but I have never been successful. It does appear that the physical state brought forth by tai chi chuan and chi gong, the seemingly slow-motion movements you have probably seen older Asian men and women practicing in the park, and which have begun to be popular among Westerners, is the relaxation response. Dr. Huang Guozhi of the Sun Yat-sen University of Medical Sciences in Guangzhou, China, did report that chi gong elicited physiologic changes consistent with the relaxation response. Still, I do not know whether this so-called energy is related to the healing abilities described in this book, but I do believe that a combination of remembered wellness and the relaxation response is involved.

Other than the physiologic changes I had already reported, I could not track the source of the energy people described, nor could I say whether they projected a feeling of spirituality onto the experience. Often, all that people could say about the experience was that it felt inherently sacred to them. They could not always say what came first—the physical or emotional reaction. And knowing something about how the brain works—that emotion is an organic contributor to mental function, and thus physical function—it makes sense that the sensations are intertwined and that people cannot distinguish between the two. Again, people seemed to be disposed to call upon belief in a higher power for soothing physical effects.

Mysticism Common to Us All

Karen Armstrong, who for seven years was a Roman Catholic nun before obtaining a degree from Oxford University, has written a scholarly and immensely popular book, *A History of God: The 4,000-Year Quest of Judaism, Christianity and Islam*. In it, she traces this common spiritual experience brought on by "silent contemplation," a method that she showed has been used by diverse religious communities for millennia. Armstrong calls the experience of God that silent contemplation engenders "mystical" because unlike the reading of scripture and other reason-based forms of worship, this experience is intuitive and nonverbal. The presence of God one might feel during silent contemplation is more mystical, much less distinct or identifiable, because "words" and theologies are not imposed upon this experience. She writes:

> The mystical experience of God has certain characteristics [that] are common to all faiths. It is a subjective experience that involves an interior journey, not a perception of an objective fact outside the self; it is undertaken through the image-making part of the mind—often called imagination—rather than

through the more cerebral, logical faculty. Finally, it is something that the mystic creates in himself or herself deliberately: certain physical or mental exercises yield the final vision; it does not always come upon them unawares.

The "physical or mental exercises" Armstrong is describing have already been scientifically documented. They are none other than the steps that elicit the physiologic relaxation response as combined with a person's heartfelt beliefs. I hypothesize that "the mystical experience common to all faiths" that Armstrong describes is the same experience my colleagues and I have identified in our patients who felt "the presence of an energy or force that seemed close to them."

The commonality of spiritual experiences and their physical manifestations, over and above the effects of remembered wellness and the relaxation response, both puzzled and excited me. It also reminded me of a paper I had written for a religion course while an undergraduate student at Wesleyan University in Connecticut. The arrogance of youth leaps out at me now, so many decades and life experiences later, for I entitled the paper, "Does God Exist?"

For the assignment, I read William James's *Varieties of Religious Experience,* a book that proved momentous to me. James argued that people of every culture and land have common experiences, worshipping a supreme or holy being. Largely as a result of reading James, I concluded in my paper that either mass mental illness pervades every society and every geography, or that this experience of God, the experience of a deity by whatever name it is called, is universal.

Nearly twenty years later, I found myself reconsidering this paper. But given that 80 percent of my patients chose prayer for their elicitation, given that a fourth of my patients described an experience of God or spirituality, and given that this experience translated into remarkable improvements in health in that group of patients, I felt the implications of my college hypotheses more deeply. Could religion really be as good for us as theologians all along had been saying it was?

God's Wellness?

Presumably, the expectancy of God's help works in the same way as does the expectancy of help from a medication, procedure, or caregiver. So asserts Dr. Jeffrey S. Levin of Eastern Virginia Medical School in his 1994 article in the journal *Social Science and Medicine*:

> The mere belief that religion or God is health enhancing may be enough to produce salutatory effects. That is, significant associations between measures of religion and health . . . may in part present evidence akin to the placebo effect. Various scriptures promise health and healing to the faithful, and the physiological effects of expectant beliefs such as this are now being documented by mind-body researchers.

The scriptures do promise healing. The word "heal" derives from an Old Saxon word meaning "whole," and for millennia, a "whole" person has been a person who demonstrated faith. Take, for example, the numerous healings reported in the Bible. Mark 5:25–34 and Luke 8:43–48 contain accounts of a woman who had bled for twelve years but when she merely touched Christ's cloak she was healed of her affliction. When Jesus turned to see who had touched his garb, he said, "Daughter, thy *faith* hath made thee whole; go in peace." Similarly, ten lepers are cleansed in Luke 17:12–19 and rush off to show examiners their condition. Only one returns to Jesus to give thanks for being cured—an act that leads Christ to remark, "Arise, go thy way: thy *faith* hath made thee whole."

On the side of the road into Jericho, a blind man begs for mercy, a cry that falls on the deaf ears of passers-by except for Jesus, who commands the man to come near. In Luke 18:42, Jesus says, "Receive thy sight; thy *faith* hath saved thee." And in Acts 14:9, one of Jesus' disciples, Paul, hears the pleas of a man in Lystra who has been crippled from birth and has never walked. "Perceiving that he had *faith* to be healed," Paul told the man to stand upright on his feet, and the man leapt up and walked (all italics added by author).

What the Gospel authors imply is clear: faith heals and makes the body whole. In his book *The Uncommon Touch*, author Tom Harpur says, "A study of the gospel reveals it is ultimately entirely about healing." And the Gospels are not alone in acclaiming faith's power. In the Holy Qur'an, we find, "And I heal the blind and the leprous, and bring the dead to life with Allah's permission and I inform you of what you should eat and what you should store in your houses; most surely there is a sign in this for you, if you are believers."

A priest who reviewed the faith healings at Lourdes, the famed Roman Catholic shrine in France, once said that people are mistaken if they think that "miracles produce faith." Quite the opposite, he says, "faith produces miracles." One of the fathers of modern American medicine seemed to agree when he went on the record proclaiming the importance of faith in healing. Dr. William Osler, first at Johns Hopkins University and later the Regis Professor of Medicine at Oxford University, wrote in 1910, "Faith in St. Johns Hopkins, as we used to call him, an atmosphere of optimism, and cheerful nurses, worked just the same sort of cures as did Aesculapeus at Epidaurus" (Aesculapeus was the ancient Roman god of medicine and healing). No matter what God was invoked, according to Dr. Osler, the cures were the same.

The Relaxation Response and Clergy Members

To follow up on the health benefits that arose from the combination of remembered wellness and the relaxation response, I began to study the faith factor in many different patients and faith communities around the world. Underwritten by Mr. Rockefeller, as I mentioned before, my colleagues and I sponsored a series of conferences in which ministers, rabbis, priests, nuns, and leaders of various religious organizations and theological schools were introduced to the prayerful applications of the relaxation response and its therapeutic effects.

At the request of Mr. Rockefeller, whose family has long supported the Memorial Sloan-Kettering Cancer Medical Center in New York City, our first clergy conference was held for its chaplains and other members of the pastoral care department. The most striking aspect of this first conference, and indeed of others thereafter, was how much these ministers needed the balm and rejuvenation that was brought forth in the relaxation response. By and large, these religious leaders, representing a variety of denominations and creeds, had this in common: they were overworked and underpaid, their jobs were very stressful, and they often had no one to turn to for their own counseling or support. Again and again, the clergy at the conference told us that their jobs were so consuming that they had abandoned their personal devotional time. Most had even stopped praying! These clergy members were elated to rediscover prayer, and to learn of the added benefits of prayers said in such a way as to evoke the relaxation response.

We went on to hold eight other Laurance Rockefeller–sponsored clergy conferences, targeting leaders of theological schools and seminaries who could teach these precepts in their diverse venues and share the news—that mind and body, East and West, scientific medicine and religion are closely related. The trickle-down effect is working, as these initial contacts have influenced religious leaders to incorporate our findings into church sermons and seminary curricula. Eventually, I began to lecture regularly at Andover Newton Theological School in Newton, Massachusetts, where I am now a part-time faculty member.

I learned a great deal from clergy members who minister to hospital patients. But Dr. Babinksy, the director of pastoral care whom I mentioned earlier, came to one of the early clergy conferences because he'd noticed a trend—that patients he visited regularly seemed to get better faster than other patients. "I could tell their complexions were rosier, and they handled the surgery or the treatment they were facing in better ways," he explains.

As a Protestant minister, Dr. Babinsky remembers being nervous about broaching the issue of meditation with patients. "It was so seemingly radical. As a Protestant chaplain, I was never sure whether patients wanted traditional prayer—I did *that* with considerable fear and trepidation. The traditions of meditation had really been lost to Christianity, although Catholic priests had more comfort with it because they had always had the centering prayer."

But Dr. Babinsky's fears quickly subsided when he saw the way that patients took to the elicitation of the relaxation response. It quells anxiety and conquers fears so that he can work with patients on "their will to live." Dr. Babinsky explains, "When patients are diagnosed or hospitalized, it's initially very traumatic and they're in a very fragile psychological state. Any small setback seems enormous to them. So they need help reframing the situation."

Ancient Meditation Techniques

While clergypeople were finding new value in prayer thanks to the relaxation response, I began cultivating relationships with the Buddhist Tibetan monks in India's Himalayan mountains, whose lifelong practice of meditation made them excellent subjects for my investigations. My colleagues and I have made four expeditions to study the Tibetan monks, most recently in 1988. Accounts of the first three expeditions and my early meetings with His Holiness the Dalai Lama can be found in my books *Beyond the Relaxation Response* and *Your Maximum Mind.* For example, our teams documented that monks could indeed dry icy, wet sheets on their naked bodies in temperatures of 40 degrees Fahrenheit. Within three to five minutes of applying the dripping three-by-six-foot sheets to their skin, the sheets began to steam! Within thirty to forty minutes, the sheets were completely dry, and they were able to repeat this process two more times.

In another observation, our team traveled to the Hemis and Gotsang monasteries in Ladakh, which are perched on the most incredible precipices at 17,500 feet above sea level. There, monks covered only by thin wool shawls and wearing only sandals on their feet spent the night of February 5, 1985, at 19,000 feet in zero and subzero temperatures. They were comfortably sustained by heat generated by their practice of g Tum-mo yoga, "fierce woman," or heat yoga. Practitioners elicit the relaxation response and then visualize themselves as having an inner channel passing from the center of their skulls through their torsos through which a heat drawn from the universe can travel, burning away defilements and improper thinking. In the same way a fierce woman protects her young, this heat burns away defilements to achieve purity.

Our Sikkim Expedition

In 1988, our team was to return to Ladakh on the eastern fringe of the Tibetan plateau to try to document the effects of the energy that allowed the monks to generate sufficient heat to survive in such extreme circumstances. The expedition was preceded by years of meticulous planning. We obtained funding from organizations including the American Institute of American Studies and the Fetzer Institute, were granted permission from the monastery and particular monks, and received the continued support of His Holiness the Dalai Lama. But when we arrived in New Delhi for our two-week mission, with forty pieces of luggage containing medical and camping equipment, we learned that the leader of the Ladakh monastery had just died, and that the monks would not allow themselves to be studied without the approval of a new leader, who had yet to be appointed.

We quickly tried to salvage our mission upon learning of another group of monks who performed the same kind of yoga at a Rumtek monastery in Sikkim, a small, previously independent kingdom between the Indian states of Assam and Nepal. Then, only by way of bullheaded persistence, remarkable good luck, and a bounty of well-wishers and quickly made friends with considerable political influence, from Dr. Phillip E. Schambra, scientific attaché of the United States embassy in New Delhi, to the Indian ministers of education and of culture, did we overcome enormous odds and secure permission to go immediately to Sikkim. This was a restricted area because it was where the Chinese previously invaded India in a 1962 border dispute. Entry to the area is only occasionally granted to tourists and travelers, who ordinarily need to apply at least six months ahead of time.

After this seemingly impossible permission had been granted in just a matter of days, India Airlines made special arrangements for us to fly to the military airport in Bagdura, from which we drove seven hours, braving treacherous mountain roads with sheer drops of two thousand feet off the side. The roads were so narrow that the bus company hired men to lean slightly out the bus window to watch and ensure that an opposite-lane bus did not come so close as to shear off a side mirror. We made this nerve-racking journey all in the hopes that the Sikkim monks, with whom we had had no previous contact, would let us watch and make measurements of their g Tum-mo yoga.

When we finally reached the monastery, we met with the chief monks, were given the traditional Tibetan tea, flavored with salt and yak butter, and were told that our trip had been in vain. Our translator, a representative of the Dalai Lama, Ven. Karma Gelek Yuthok, relayed that the monks no longer performed the ritual of drying wet sheets and that they did not want to be observed in their sacred meditations.

That night we ate dinner—hard-boiled eggs and peanut butter and jelly sandwiches—while sitting on earthen floors in the refuse-strewn room of the monastery guest house. Each of us nursed disappointment that after so many years of planning and after overcoming recent travails, the expedition had proven so fruitless. But before we went to sleep, one of the monks with whom we had met, Ven. Bakar Rinpoche, came to us and agreed to be studied, an act that led two other monks, Lama Chonyl Dondup and Lama Gyaltsen, to acquiesce as well.

So we finally got to do what we had come all this way to accomplish—measure the vital signs of these men who were employing ancient Tibetan meditation to elicit the relaxation response with which we were so familiar. During their meditation, we discovered they experienced outlandishly low rates of oxygen consumption or metabolism. While patients we had measured in Boston experienced an average 10 to 17 percent drop in metabolism from the relaxation response, Bakar Rinpoche experienced a decrease of 64 percent—the lowest level ever documented in a human being. I had often heard reports about Indian yogis who survived hours of being buried alive, and although the Sikkim monks did not perform such acts, we now knew how humans might survive the ritual. The yogis could sustain themselves by lowering their metabolism dramatically enough to extract sufficient oxygen from the loose soil around them.

Superhuman Feats

Indeed, having documented the mind-boggling physical feats that the monks performed by way of the faith factor, I was curious about how far faith might go. With such a strong faith propelling believers, and channeled through proven mental focusing techniques, I wondered if other "superhuman" stunts were possible. On other expeditions, my colleagues and I tried to confirm legendary reports that Tibetan monks levitate, rising and hovering above the ground during meditation. But when we were allowed to view the levitation of monks in the mountain hamlet of Chail, it appeared only to be an act of considerable physical agility in which monks, leg-locked in lotus position, sprang several inches off the floor. They did not hover. When I asked a chief monk whether hovering was possible, I was told through a translator that the sages of old had done so. When I asked, "Is it possible today?" the monk replied, with a twinkle in his eye, "There is no need. Today we have airplanes."

I don't believe it is possible to hover or to perform other physical feats that defy Newtonian physics. Don't get me wrong, the faith factor is a remarkable feature of human physiology. The mind is certainly capable of incredible influence over physiology, as we've seen in the Tibetan monks in India. In fact, many athletes draw upon the faith factor during competition and experience the exhilaration that comes with being "in the zone." A tennis player quoted in *The New York Times* once described the zone as "so complete and intense that it evokes a state of almost semiconscious euphoria—one that many believe bears a resemblance to hypnosis, and enables a top player to achieve his or her peak performance."

Sports psychologists say that athletes in the zone experience great happiness, a sense of timelessness, effortlessness, and positive thinking. They often *expect* to win. The retired tennis great Chris Evert Lloyd confirmed this, saying, "You play in the zone, over your head where everything is like a dream. When you play matches like that, you want to play more."

Peak Experiences

This is very similar to the "peak" or religious experiences that people sometimes ascribe to meditation or prayer. I've always found it difficult to pin down what people are talking about when they refer to peak experiences. But Dr. Stanley R. Dean, professor of psychiatry at the Universities of Miami and Florida, captured what I mean when I refer to peak experiences when he wrote that they "produce a superhuman transmutation of consciousness that defies description. The mind, divinely intoxicated, literally reels and trips over itself, groping and struggling for words of sufficient exultation and grandeur to portray the transcendental vision. As yet we have no adequate words."

You may recall from the previous chapter that I discourage patients from expecting peak experiences—inwardly and outwardly dramatic effects that are often associated with intense prayer or meditation. It is, I have explained, defeatist to expect fireworks because those expectations will interfere with the focus needed to bring about the relaxation response.

This is often a difficult message to get across to people because our society is captivated by encounters with God and immortality, and we are particularly intrigued by the idea that the divine articulates itself in fantastic and conspicuous ways. In revivals and worship services, in motivational groups and mind-over-matter seminars, people faint and convulse, froth at the mouth, speak in tongues, handle poisonous snakes, walk over fiery coals, and claim to levitate. We hear accounts in which people feel climactically reborn, see Madonna statues cry, or are summoned by the voice of God, Satan, or a deceased relative with an important message.

In my twenty-five-year study of patients eliciting the relaxation response, I have found that experiences this dramatic are relatively rare. While the unusual and awesome are possible, it appears that a broad spectrum of peaceful and exhilarating sensations are facilitated by the relaxation response, many of which defy precise description, a portion of which seem to transcend daily human experience and feel spiritual in nature. All of these experiences, mild through fantastic, appear to be equally physiologically healing.

In a world that craves them, it's wonderful to know that sacred and spiritual experiences of all kinds, some peak but most simply peaceful and restorative, are within our grasp. As I noted, the November 28, 1994, *Newsweek* reported that outside of church, 45 percent of Americans sense the sacred during meditation, whereas 68 percent have that sense at the birth of a child, and 26 percent during sex. This survey makes it clear that sacred experiences are very accessible in life.

Because of the way in which our brains are wired, and the faith factor that maximizes the relaxation response, I began to understand that the spirituality our world so ardently desires dwells within us and is relatively easily called forth. If it is your desire, you can apply your religious beliefs to elicit the relaxation response and flex what may seem to you to be a kind of spiritual muscle. Whatever your beliefs, when you elicit the relaxation response, you'll be flexing a mind/body mechanism that has proven physiologic merit as well.

CHAPTER 8

FAITH
HEALS

In her book *A History of God*, Karen Armstrong tells the story of a group of Jews in the Auschwitz concentration camp who decide, one afternoon, to put God on trial. God is brought up on charges of cruelty and betrayal and the arguments for and against God begin. Despite believing that God is supposed to counter evil and serve as a comfort to humans, this impromptu death camp court finds no evidence of divine intervention in their horrific world nor any extenuating circumstances that relieve God of culpability. The rabbi announces the verdict: God is guilty as charged and, presumably, worthy of death. But then the rabbi glances up at those assembled and says that the trial has concluded. It is, he tells them, time for the evening prayer.

We saw in the last chapter how natural it was for people to combine remembered wellness and the relaxation response in a merger I call the faith factor. I found that my patients got accustomed to this type of prayer almost as if it were second nature to them. I began to look for more evidence that faith was as intractable and as powerful in human physiology as these initial investigations had suggested. I turned to the medical literature to find the evidence which existed that spirituality and religious life are good for people. These findings are the substance of this chapter.

Faith Throughout History

I quickly learned that there is not a civilization known to us that did not have faith in God or gods. For millennia, faith has enjoyed relevance to all the world's people, but when the West began to divide the mind/body spheres, sending faith and reason to opposite corners, faith did not appear to fare as well as reason because it became a private, personal matter, and reason became a public, promotable good. The battles for terrain have often been bitter, as Martin Luther amply demonstrated, saying, "Reason is the greatest enemy that faith has; it never comes to the aid of spiritual things, but—more frequently than not—struggles against the divine Word, treating with contempt all that emanates from God."

So much human potential has been squandered in this standoff. Scientists have had contempt for God, rarely making religious faith the focus of scientific study. Dr. Robert D. Orr and the Reverend George Isaac of the University of Chicago reported in their review of seven major American primary care journals that of 1,066 articles, only twelve—a mere 1.1 percent—of them assessed religious considerations. Of all the features and characteristics of patients that could be and were studied, religion and faith were almost completely ignored.

In another excellent review, Dr. Levin and Dr. Preston L. Schiller, also of Eastern Virginia Medical School, surveyed over two hundred studies conducted over the last two hundred years in which religious findings *were* assessed in English language medical journals. But to think that in two hundred years, only two hundred of the hundreds of thousands of English medical journal articles even bothered to look at faith demonstrates just how taboo God has become in the recent history of Western medicine.

Dr. Levin explains that "Western biomedicine, of which epidemiology is a part, is still wrestling with a body-mind dualism that defies consensus; thus for most epidemiologists any resolution of a body-mind-spirit pluralism is simply beyond consideration." And Dr. Levin concludes, "As a result, the idea that one's religious background of experiences might in some way influence one's health has remained part of the folklore of discussion on the fringes of the research community."

But this is slowly changing. Scientists are now more actively mining older research for evidence, and newer studies are being launched. And just as was true in my review of research into remembered wellness, the evidence that does exist on the health benefits of faith were very convincing. In one of the most important summaries, Dr. Levin reviewed hundreds of epidemiologic studies to conclude that belief in God lowers death rates and increases health. And in 1995, Dr. Thomas E. Oxman and his colleagues at Dartmouth Medical School reported that heart disease patients over the age of fifty-five who had had open-heart surgery for either coronary artery or aortic valve disease, and who had received solace and comfort from their religious beliefs, were three times more likely to survive than those who did not.

In most scientific studies done in the past, researchers focused on the benefits of participation in organized religion. They undoubtedly did so because participation was easier to measure than belief. And yet, by excluding patients with less publicly practiced religious beliefs, they presumed that those beliefs were not influential. But as research into less publicly practiced beliefs in God has begun to accumulate, the outcomes have turned out to be the same. My review of the research reveals that regardless of how traditional one's practice of religious beliefs, whenever faith is present, remembered wellness is triggered and health can be improved.

Health and Religious Commitment

According to a 1990 Gallup poll, 95 percent of Americans say they believe in God and 76 percent say they pray on a regular basis. And in a comprehensive and impressive review of the scientific literature on the medical effects of spiritual experiences, Dr. Dale A. Matthews, Dr. David B. Larson, and Ms. Constance P. Barry have found evidence that religious factors have a widespread, profound influence on health (see Table 6). In their scholarly synthesis, *The Faith Factor: An Annotated Bibliography of Clinical Research on Spiritual Subjects*, they found that religious factors were involved with increased survival; reduced alcohol, cigarette, and drug use; reduced anxiety, depression, and anger; reduced blood pressure; and improved quality of life for patients with cancer and heart disease.

In one interesting experiment performed by Dr. Peter Pressman of Northwestern University Medical School and his colleagues, thirty elderly women recovering from surgical corrections of their broken hips were studied to assess the relationship between their religious beliefs and their medical and

TABLE 6

THE INFLUENCE OF

RELIGIOUS FACTORS ON HEALTH*

CONDITION	NUMBER OF STUDIES	NUMBER OF STUDIES IN WHICH HEALTHFUL EFFECTS WERE PRESENT	PERCENT IN WHICH HEALTHFUL EFFECTS WERE PRESENT
Reduced Alcohol Use	18	16	89
Reduced Nicotine Use	6	6	100
Reduced Drug Use	12	12	100
Improved Psychological Symptoms Including Adjustment and Coping	15	14	93
Reduced Depression	17	12	71

*Data summarized from: D. A. Matthews, D. B. Larson, and C. P. Barry, *The Faith Factor: An Annotated Bibliography of Clinical Research on Spiritual Subjects.* Vol. 1. (John Templeton Foundation, 1994).

psychiatric health. Those with strong religious beliefs were able to walk significantly farther and were less likely to be depressed. Even if the patients walked farther because they were less depressed, the outcome is nevertheless impressive.

Religious commitment is consistently associated with better health. The greater a person's commitment, the fewer his or her psychological symptoms, the better his or her general health, the lower the blood pressure, and the longer the survival. Across the board, in groups of different ages, ethnicities, and religions,

TABLE 6 *(continued)*

THE INFLUENCE OF
RELIGIOUS FACTORS ON HEALTH

CONDITION	NUMBER OF STUDIES	NUMBER OF STUDIES IN WHICH HEALTHFUL EFFECTS WERE PRESENT	PERCENT IN WHICH HEALTHFUL EFFECTS WERE PRESENT
Reduced Hostility	4	4	100
Reduced General Anxiety	11	8	73
Reduced Death Anxiety	15	10	67
Improved General Health	5	4	80
Reduced Blood Pressure	5	4	80
Improved Quality of Life in Cancer Patients	8	7	88
Improved Quality of Life in Heart Disease Patients	6	4	67
Increased Survival	9	8	89

among patients with very different diseases and conditions, religious commitment brings with it a lifetime of benefits.

Religion usually promotes healthy lifestyles and behaviors. Among others, Mormons and Seventh-Day Adventists dissuade their members from smoking, drinking, or having extramarital sex (which is associated with a greater risk of sexually transmitted diseases) and encourage healthful diets and exercise. Seventh-Day Adventists, who discourage tobacco and alcohol use, have substantially lower rates of cancer—especially lung, bladder, and colon cancer—when compared to the general population, even compared to those who abstain from alcohol use. These religious practitioners, as well as clergy members of all faiths, are mentally and physically healthier than average Americans.

Religious people consistently report greater life satisfaction, marital satisfaction, well-being, altruism, and self-esteem than do nonreligious people (see Table 7). Given everything we know about both remembered wellness and about the impact of stress and turmoil on our health, the happiness and contentment engendered by faith proves an extraordinary contributor to health.

In twenty-two of twenty-seven studies, attendance at religious services was correlated with better health. Worship services are full of potentially therapeutic elements—music, aesthetic surroundings, familiar rituals, prayer and contemplation, distraction from everyday tensions, the opportunity for socializing and fellowship, and education.

TABLE 7
THE INFLUENCE OF RELIGIOUS FACTORS ON PSYCHOLOGICAL MEASUREMENTS*

PSYCHOSOCIAL MEASUREMENT	NUMBER OF STUDIES	NUMBER OF STUDIES IN WHICH POSITIVE EFFECTS WERE PRESENT	PERCENT IN WHICH POSITIVE EFFECTS WERE PRESENT
Greater Life Satisfaction	13	12	92
Greater Marital Satisfaction	3	3	100
Greater Well-being	16	15	94
Greater Altruism	5	3	60
Greater Self-esteem	4	2	50

*Data summarized from: D. A. Matthews, D. B. Larson, and C. P. Barry, *The Faith Factor: An Annotated Bibliography of Clinical Research on Spiritual Subjects.* Vol. 1. (John Templeton Foundation, 1994).

The Religious Ritual

Remembered wellness makes the religious ritual a very powerful mechanism. There is something very influential about invoking a ritual that you may first have practiced in childhood, about regenerating the neural pathways that were formed in your youthful experience of faith. In my medical practice, this has proven true, even, I might add, among many adults who have rejected the religion they practiced in their youth. Even if you experience the ritual from an entirely different perspective of maturity and life history, the words you read, the songs you sing, and the prayers you invoke will soothe you in the same way they did in what was perhaps a simpler time in your life. Even if you don't consciously appreciate that there is any real drama or emotion attached to the ritual, the brain retains a memory of the constellation of activities associated with the ritual, both the emotional content that allows the brain to weigh its importance and the nerve cell firings, interactions, and chemical releases that were first activated.

As long as I have been teaching people the relaxation response, encouraging patients to personalize focusing techniques by adopting words, prayers, phrases, or mantras that are meaningful to them, I never fail to be impressed by the impact of familiar rituals. Years ago, Sally Nash, a benefactor of the Mind/Body Medical Institute even though she had never actually used the facility herself, developed ovarian cancer. The woman absolutely refused to believe that cancer would be her downfall, ignoring for a period of some months the treatments mainstream medicine could offer her—drugs and procedures, two legs of the three-legged stool I maintain are needed to optimize health. Instead, she embarked on a strict macrobiotic diet and practiced the relaxation response faithfully. But eventually her bowels became obstructed because of metastatic malignant tumors, and I demanded, both as her doctor and her friend, that she have surgery immediately to relieve the blockage. Without the operation, she

would surely have died. But despite the grim prognosis, Ms.
Nash only reluctantly agreed to the operation and then only
on one condition: that I be with her when she went to the hospital and received the anesthesia.

Of course I readily agreed. Later that afternoon, we were
together in the anteroom at the Deaconess Hospital in Boston
where she was to be given anesthesia and prepared for the operation. The anesthesiologist who came into the room was
massive, the size and stature of a football player, his demeanor
quiet and businesslike. Already masked, he and I acknowledged one another and he indicated he was ready to give Ms.
Nash the anesthesia for the operation. She asked me to hold
her hand and to take her through the steps of the relaxation
response, using the same recitation she had been using—the
beginning of the 23rd Psalm, "The Lord is my shepherd."

As the anesthesiologist began the anesthesia drip, I repeated out loud along with her quiet recitation, "The Lord is
my shepherd . . . The Lord is my shepherd . . . The Lord is my
shepherd" on each of her outbreaths until eventually the
anesthesia took effect and she lost consciousness. When I
looked up, the anesthesiologist—whom I'd likened to Dick
Butkus just moments before—was softly shaking, his mask
soaked with tears. For the woman herself, the recitation of a
familiar psalm with a doctor she trusted was a deep source of
calm. But the ritual also carried with it power that I could not
have predicted, eliciting in this straightforward, dutiful anesthesiologist a profound emotional response.

Author Karen Armstrong also heralds the importance of religious rituals, writing:

> Many of the people who attend religious services in
> our society are not interested in theology, want noth-
> ing too exotic and dislike the idea of change. They
> find the established rituals provide them with a link
> with tradition and give them a sense of security. They
> do not expect brilliant ideas from the sermon and
> are disturbed by changes in the liturgy. In rather the
> same way, many of the pagans of the late antiquity

loved to worship the ancestral gods, as generations had done before them. The old rituals gave them a sense of identity, celebrated local traditions and seemed an assurance that things would continue as they were.

This is, of course, why changes in liturgy are so wrenching to parishioners. Even if the rituals seem formal and antiquated to modern thinking, they are mysterious and awe-evoking and leave indelible marks on our brains. For this reason, I have found that many of my Catholic patients, those who have experienced a ritual-laden religion, are quick to embrace the relaxation response. If they are so inclined, I encourage them to say their rosary or prayer in the language in which they first learned or heard it, be it in Latin or Spanish, Italian or another language. Despite the fact that they now predominantly speak English, recalling a native tongue produces a special reverence and helps ensure adherence to the practice.

This may also be an important lesson to other religious communities trying to maintain the delicate balance between ritual and innovation, retaining meaningful traditions while shedding practices that are outdated or unappealing. While religious rites are particularly stirring, patriotic and other secular traditions work the same way, the brain retaining from childhood a visceral, active memory of the songs, symbols, words, and gestures so that the body is invigorated and nourished when they are remembered.

Fellowship

The fellowship offered to people in their religious communities is equally restorative. According to Dr. Levin, the history of epidemiological studies suggests that the social support, sense of belonging, and convivial fellowship engendered by religion "serve to buffer the adverse effects of stress and anger, perhaps via psychoneuroimmunologic pathways." He speculates that religious involvement "may trigger a multifactorial sequence of biological processes leading to better health."

Of course there are many other routes of receiving social support and fellowship than in religious circles. But religion does represent an important source of socializing for many, and in a study reported in the *American Journal of Epidemiology* of nearly seven thousand men and women between the age of thirty and sixty-nine in Alameda County, California, researchers found that social isolation has pervasive health consequences. Higher degrees of social connection consistently relate to decreased mortality, whether the connection is fueled by family and friends, by group membership or church involvement. This very important finding by Dr. Lisa F. Berkman of Yale University and Dr. Leonard S. Syme of the University of California, Berkeley, established that death rates, a clear and unambiguous measurement, were influenced by levels of social support.

Jean-Paul Sartre once said that hell is other people. But at least when it comes to our physical health, our ability to overcome disease and to live longer, people truly need other people. Medicine has long appreciated that married people enjoy better health than single, divorced, or widowed people. For more than a decade, scientists at the University of Michigan studied 2,754 people in the Tecumseh, Michigan, area and found that men who did less volunteer work, who had less social contact, and who were relatively sedentary were significantly more likely to die during the course of the study than men who volunteered regularly and had more social contact.

And in an often-quoted study, Dr. David Spiegel and co-workers at Stanford University School of Medicine and University of California, Berkeley, demonstrated that upon assessments ten years after treatment, women with breast cancer who participated in support groups lived eighteen months longer on average than women who did not. In the Dartmouth Medical School study of patients undergoing heart surgery that I referred to above, the patients who participated in community and social groups, like those who received solace from their religious beliefs, were three times more likely to survive. But those who participated in both social activities and received solace from their religious faith had a tenfold increase in survival!

Still, hospitals and clinics cannot supply their communities with the plethora of opportunities for social encounters and support sponsored by most churches and religious organizations. Be it weekly church or synagogue services, daily masses or temples devoted to prayer several times each day, be it Bible study or bingo night, confirmation classes, preparation for bar mitzvah or bat mitzvah, potluck suppers or youth groups, marriage encounter weekends or church camps, Sunday school or soup kitchens, religious institutions ensure that their members get ample doses, not just of faith but of healthy social interactions.

Altruism

Traditional religion has always encouraged believers to help others, to be altruistic, to tithe, and to spread the good word. But in the process of sharing the wealth, believers also garner better health.

My friend Allan Luks, whom I met when he was executive director of the Institute for the Advancement of Health, now serves as executive director of Big Brothers/Big Sisters of New York City. Luks devoted a book to documenting *The Healing Power of Doing Good.* In a survey of thousands of volunteers across the nation, Luks discovered that people who help other people consistently report better health than peers in their age group. Many also say that their health markedly improved when they began volunteer work.

Luks calls this phenomenon "the helper's high." Ninety-five percent of those he surveyed indicated that helping others on a regular, personal basis gives them a physical, good sensation. Nine out of ten identified specific characteristics of the physical sensation or rush, including a sudden warmth, increased energy, and a sense of euphoria. They also reported long-term effects of greater calm and relaxation.

Not only does the act of doing good bring about this helper's high, eight out of ten of the volunteers surveyed said the health benefits returned when they later remembered the helping act (i.e., remembered wellness). It's important to note that the overall rewards noted in Luks's survey were reaped from helping strangers, not just family and friends. Although the causes were diverse, the selfless act of helping others always resulted in enhanced health, making altruism a viable form of self-care.

Intercessory Prayer and Therapeutic Touch

Some studies indicate that intercessory prayer, that is, praying for someone else, is effective, although further research is needed. However, it is interesting to see that intercessory prayer may have worked in the following study because the patients did not know anyone was praying for their recovery. Thus, if the intercessory prayers worked, it could not have been the result of remembered wellness. Almost four hundred patients who had once been hospitalized in a San Francisco coronary care unit were studied for ten months. Half of the patients were assigned someone to pray on their behalf while the other half were not. The patients who had received intercessory prayer had significantly fewer episodes of congestive heart failure, fewer cardiac arrests, less pneumonia, and required fewer diuretics and antibiotics.

Religious congregations have long featured prayer chains and lay leaders who visited hospitalized parishioners but, with news spreading about the physical benefits of the relaxation response, prayer and "the laying on of hands" have become far more serious endeavors. Nurses have now adapted the religious tradition of the laying on of hands in a field called "therapeutic touch"—found to significantly decrease postoperative pain, to decrease patients' needs for analgesia, and in one study, to decrease headache pain in 90 percent of patients with tension headaches. Doctors discovered that wound-healing rates were significantly improved when therapeutic touch was used, and other investigators demonstrated that hospitalized patients treated with the therapy experienced a significant reduction in anxiety.

Therapeutic touch practitioners claim to transmit an energy that I discussed in the previous chapter, and the treatment may or may not involve actual physical touch of a patient. Meditative in stance when they care for patients, practitioners believe that even if actual contact is not made, their healing energy field connects with patients.

Again, as I said before, I have not been able to verify the existence of energy fields in my scientific endeavors. But I do believe that remembered wellness is at work in therapeutic touch. And additionally, in cases where actual physical contact is made, patients may be benefiting from what I believe will eventually be the scientifically established healing effects of human touch. I've often heard patients remark about how much it meant to them that a surgeon or anesthesiologist held their hand when they were losing consciousness with anesthesia. And we know that babies who are denied holding and affection in their formative first months suffer long-term effects of this deprivation of touch. Later in the book, I'll make some distinctions between conventional and unconventional medicine, but for now, suffice it to say that I believe that science will go on to find inherent healing value in human touch and that this could redeem the value of unconventional medicine's therapies that include massage.

My Attempts to Quantify Faith Healing

More than a decade ago, I decided to study a self-described "healer." In the past, I had been approached by various healers who, after reading *The Relaxation Response*, believed they evoked the relaxation response when they performed their healings. As fascinated as I was by their claims, I was always hesitant to start such studies, worried that I might take my interests in remembered wellness too far and jeopardize my credibility in the field. But Lady Raeburn (Addy), a former Olympic skier for Great Britain, the wife of the former governor of H.M. Tower of London and the descendant of a distinguished line of British naval officers (incidentally a distant relative of the former U.S. World War II admiral William "Bull" Halsey), was touring the United States with her husband when she made an appointment to see me and to ask me to study her healing power. As the wife of a prominent politician, Lady Raeburn assured me that if I were to engage in these studies, she could and would keep our work secret.

Lady Raeburn told me that she first noticed her healing ability when she was seventeen years old and could calm an aunt in the throes of a persistent and violent "nervous breakdown." Later, while skiing, she broke a bone in her lower leg and helped heal herself, drawing upon her healing resources and those of another self-described healer. She went on to heal animals and then fellow athletes who suffered broken limbs. And in time, she began healing people with a wide range of disorders.

If I was willing, Lady Raeburn said, she would donate her time and fly back and forth from London to be tested. We agreed to pursue some experiments, promising that mum would be the word if nothing significant emerged from our findings.

I found a laboratory at Harvard Medical School that honored our requests for discretion. I hypothesized that if such a healer could influence simpler life forms—animals that didn't have highly developed nervous systems, or plants—it might be possible to establish the existence of a healer's "energy." If it existed, this energy had to be shown to have effects distinct from those of remembered wellness, and since what Lady Raeburn practiced was the laying on of hands, I could think of no experiment with humans that would be free of beliefs.

We began our experiments with kernels of corn that sprout very quickly in water. I had, essentially, poisoned corn kernels by immersing them in dilute salt solutions to inhibit their growth. Lady Raeburn held her hands over one group of poisoned kernels, and amazingly, they did sprout more quickly than the other poisoned corn.

Next, we worked with planaria, worms that regenerate when they are cut in half. We used the eye spots as markers for a fully regenerated body. After we cut all the worms, the planaria that Lady Raeburn held her hands over regenerated more quickly, and the eye spots on the worms she "healed" appeared more rapidly than on the other worms.

These were very interesting results. But the problem was, I was never able to replicate them in a second or third round of investigations. Lady Raeburn and I have remained friends for years, despite the mystery we are unable to solve.

And while a review of the relevant literature by Dr. David J. Benor of London, England, cites effects of spiritual healing on yeast, bacteria, plants, and animals, the majority of these results have not been replicated by other investigators. And because replication proved impossible in my experiments, I am wary of these results.

Over the years, I have heard many examples of pets reacting to their owners' contemplative states when the individuals evoked the relaxation response. Over twenty years ago, the head of the Medical Department of New York Telephone, Dr. Gilbeart H. Collings, Jr., along with other colleagues and I performed a study of the effects of regular elicitation of the relaxation response on a group of AT&T operator supervisors who, at that time, handled caller complaints and suffered high degrees of stress because of it. Dr. Collings called me one day to report that he had been alerted by a number of supervisors eliciting the relaxation response that their otherwise aloof pets clamored to be near them during the practice, scratching at the door, wanting to be let into the room and to sit close, and then demonstrating unusually affectionate behavior. This same reaction has been reported to me so often over the years that I have termed the phenomenon "the St. Francis effect," recalling the legend in which St. Francis tamed the wild wolf and attracted birds and other creatures.

The St. Francis Effect

A most dramatic example of the St. Francis effect came from a woman in a group of state employees to whom I was giving a talk in Concord, New Hampshire. The woman related the story of two beautiful Egyptian geese she kept on her farm. These magnificent birds, a male and female, were, however, very ornery and aloof, at all times maintaining a healthy distance from her, never coming within a few feet of her even at feeding time. In the spring, the woman liked to practice meditation sitting by the pond on her farm. And one May day, she was doing so with her eyes closed and her meditation underway when she happened to open her eyes and saw that the two geese were right in front of her, their heads inches from her face. She was startled but closed her eyes again, returning to her meditation, and in another minute or so opened her eyes to find these beautiful animals still close at hand, this time prancing and extending their wings and legs in what seemed to her to be a kind of dance. Again the woman was amazed but she closed her eyes and continued her meditation, and minutes later felt the geese sit, one on either side of her, stretch out their necks and lay their heads across her lap. To her astonishment, she told us, the geese rested there for some time.

I have always attributed the St. Francis effect to the pheromones or scents put off by humans (and animals), which are diminished when stress is reduced and bodies are calm. It appears that when we relax, we release less of the scents that usually scare or discourage animals from coming close to us. Good veterinarians and animal trainers understand this very well. I once read that women in New York City, among the world's most harried, most exciting, and, therefore, most stress-inducing environments, use more deodorant than any other comparable population group in the country. Although we don't often think about the minute release of scents issued by our bodies when under stress, the effects are nevertheless measurable.

Dr. Larry Dossey, once an internist and now a full-time author with five books about spirituality and healing to his credit, argues that prayer is potent not only for people but for animals, plants, and lower organisms. (This might, of course, lend credence to gardeners who insist that talking to plants produces better growth.) Dr. Dossey undoubtedly welcomes additional research that I believe is required to substantiate a link between beliefs and animal and plant physiology.

The Evidence of Faith Healing

While the effects of faith on animals and plants remain in question, I do not doubt that the aura or reverence humans lend to healers evokes remembered wellness. This is not to say that we should venerate caregivers, or pepper our lives with superstitions, but we should appreciate the fact that the marvel we attach to healers and to conventional and unconventional therapies may be therapeutic in and of itself.

I also believe that there is something powerful about pilgrimages, which humans have, for centuries, believed are healing and restorative. Think of how people flock to shrines and holy sites, or travel to the Harvard teaching hospitals, Johns Hopkins Hospital, the Menninger and the Mayo Clinics. I suspect that when people make long journeys to see healers, to visit places they associate with healing, the buildup of anticipation and hope engenders a profound form of remembered wellness. Clearly, patients benefit from confidence in and even admiration for their caregivers. Indeed, there may be ways that traditional medicine and its practitioners can position themselves to better conform our practices to the instinctual and even unconscious preferences of our patients, much as the previously mentioned system of feng shui suggests.

But in this book, I am emphasizing confidence in and admiration for one's internal healing resources in hopes that we can strike a better balance between what caregivers give us or do for us—medicines and procedures—and the underappreciated role of self-care. Essentially I am offering ways in which individuals can optimize remembered wellness, given the fact that conventional medicine is just beginning to incorporate the many lessons of remembered wellness.

Even though faith and beliefs do have legitimate healing powers, "faith healing" is a term our society has come to associate with religious entrepreneurs, with those who manipulate rather than minister, with a greater concern for fund-raising than care-giving. But as society begins to embrace mind/body medicine and to grasp that remembered wellness is effective in handling the majority of medical complaints, so too must we acknowledge the legitimacy of some faith healing.

The beauty of remembered wellness is that it needs no clinical white coat; it relies on the faith of individuals, of lay persons, of people with and without specific medical knowledge, simply on the expectancies of all people. The danger, of course, is with medical practitioners and nonmedical practitioners who try to channel expectancy and belief to make a profit or aggrandize themselves.

Still, looking at what we traditionally consider faith healing, in a 1984 telephone survey of more than five hundred adults in Richmond, Virginia, researchers found that 14 percent reported they had been physically healed as a result of prayer or divine intervention. Twelve percent claimed to have been cured of colds and flus, while others claimed that emotional problems, back problems, fractures, and cancer had been assuaged or aided. There was, however, no confirmation of these claims by the researchers.

In another investigation of faith healing in Baltimore, Maryland, 67 percent claimed some positive effects on physical problems, which included back aches, chronic pain, and arthritis. For psychological problems including depression, anxiety, fear, or anger, the rate of healing was 77 percent. Again, there was no independent measure of these claims by others, but relief was, nevertheless, afforded to people who had been suffering. In one objective study performed in the Netherlands, laying on of hands yielded reports of greater patient well-being but no reduction in systolic or diastolic blood pressures.

Despite the lack of confirmation or consensus in these studies of faith healing, we know from the previously mentioned experiments on remembered wellness that a caregiver's belief can empower healing. Yet we must further study faith healing if we are to credit it for benefits over and above that of remembered wellness.

The more we learn about faith's medical prowess, the more we see mainline religious denominations returning to the healing fold. Andover Newton Theological School in Massachusetts is one of many theological schools now offering instruction in faith healing, and not just in the traditional pastoral care and chaplain programs. The seminary's previous chairman of the Department of Psychology and Clinical Studies as well as director of Clinical Pastoral Education, Dr. Henry C. Brooks, explains, "Healing was once a major part of the mission of the church but we abdicated it. We began to think that healing was a secular enterprise. But now, having become immersed in the study of mind/body connections, we realize we have a valuable role. We've become less self-conscious about it, that healing is part of the Christian tradition, that it isn't just a gimmick from a charlatan. Now faith healing is a central focus for us and we hope to be at the forefront in teaching others about it."

Mind/Body Theology

In the works, religious scholars tell me, is a full theology and religious doctrine that celebrates mind/body/soul connections and that may guide religious believers in understanding and appreciating the religious implications of these connections. Yet others are not so welcoming of the news that we physically benefit from religious beliefs, and they believe the medical findings will only undermine faith. I have heard Dr. Martin E. Marty, senior scholar at the Park Ridge Center for Health, Faith and Ethics in Chicago, say that "the next major assault to God will come from neurobiology, which will try to reduce God to neurons."

Years ago, an eminent theologian gave me some advice that helped ease my mind on this matter. When facts began to present themselves, and the faith factor began to emerge as a significant health benefit, I was worried that religious people would view my investigations as an attempt to "reduce God to neurons." I was also concerned that by trying to learn more about remembered wellness in the potent form of religious faith, it might appear that I was trying to prove or disprove the existence of God.

So I made an appointment to meet with the dean of Harvard Divinity School. Dean Krister Stendhal was, at that time, the leader of this very prestigious school of theology, which was founded in 1811. Dean Stendhal is Lutheran in orientation and imposing in stature. Despite his being very thin and stooped, the dean's presence was immense—well over six feet tall to my straight-backed five foot nine.

I sat down in the recesses of a deep-cushioned chair in front of the dean's desk and began my rehearsed statement. I told him about remembered wellness and the relaxation response. I told him how I'd first noted the physiologic changes in practitioners of Transcendental Meditation, and about the incredible feats the Tibetan monks were able to perform during meditation. I told him about the faith factor, and about patients who benefited from increased spirituality. And ultimately I told Dr. Stendhal that I was concerned my investigations might undermine the practice of religion. I needed his advice.

Dean Stendhal took in all of this before rising from his chair, slowly walking over to me, and laying a hand on my shoulder. Looming over me in my low-sitting chair, he declared, "Young man, don't worry about us. Religion and prayer were here before you and they will be here after you. You do your thing and we will do ours."

In my endeavors, I have tried not to reduce God to neurons, but to heighten medical science's respect for all beliefs, including belief in God, so that we understand how remarkably powerful is the mind/body/soul we inhabit.

The data we've presented here is undeniable. Faith is indeed central to human life and health. The painter Marc Chagall once said, "Do not leave my hand without light." My search began to persuade me that light is to the painter what faith is to humankind. More and more, I became convinced that faith and hope are our primal instincts, a kind of light to which we are naturally drawn. As did the Jewish prisoners in Auschwitz, we may reject the logic of God but we cannot deny the emotional and physical solace of spiritual life.

CHAPTER 9

WIRED
FOR GOD

Much of the time, the scientific quest I've described in this book was driven by the question "Is that all there is?" Scientific medicine always seemed to me, in the patients I encountered and in the research I compiled, to be cordoning off parts of the human experience it wanted to affect. In the process, we neglected those aspects that patients, if asked, would probably identify as the essence or meaning of their lives. This was particularly frustrating because my research consistently demonstrated that "the essence of life" was also a wellspring of health.

Acting on Instinct

But as much as my journey was pushed onward by medical research results, it was also driven by instincts. So in this chapter, I will tell you what I instinctively came to believe was timeless and immutable about human physiology and human existence. As informed as my search has been by the traditional measures of science, and as much evidence as I have that my conclusions are scientifically sound, it is at this point in my search that I've reached the end of what I believe science can ultimately prove.

Very early on in my quest for answers, nearly thirty years ago, I had one of the most profound thoughts I've ever had. Like most of my better ideas, it came to me when I was shaving. Mind and body research aside, I've found that nothing rouses the intellect like a sharp blade making tracks across one's face. So it was that I stood in front of a mirror one morning, razor to chin and deep in thought. I was mulling over the facts as I knew them at that point: Scientists had proven the existence of a brain-controlled state of relaxation in animals, the same relaxation response that I would later identify in humans.

I'd seen that Transcendental Meditation practitioners could relax the physiologic mechanisms usually aroused by stress.

And although at the time I didn't know the precise formula for calling this relaxation forward, the steps did not appear to be mysterious or difficult to learn. I hypothesized that I would be able to find examples of the use of a repetitive focus in both secular and religious settings, and speculated that the relaxation response was being elicited in everything from Lamaze breathing exercises to religious rituals around the world.

Razor in hand, I continued thinking, harking back to my college paper and the commonalties of religious experience that William James had so beautifully documented. It seemed that as long as people had lived, they had worshipped.

And then it struck me. "This is prayer!" I exclaimed to my half-shaven reflection. Perhaps this tendency of humans to worship and believe was rooted in our physiology, written into our genes, and encoded in our very makeup. Perhaps it is what distinguishes us from other life forms, this innate desire to believe and to practice our beliefs. Perhaps instinctively, human beings had always known that worshipping a higher power was good for them. And indeed, if they were calling forth the relaxation response, medical science could *prove* it was good for them! I speculated that perhaps humans are, in a profound physical way, "wired for God."

Wired for God?

The notion that humans might be wired for God seemed to me to be so beyond the realm of traditional scientific study that, as exhilarated as I was about the possibility of its being true, I was also immediately very fearful. Who was I to try to quantify and document faith in God? I could not have found any subject matter more controversial. There was nothing more sacred to people than religious faith. And there was nothing so "unscientific" as faith. Moreover, I felt woefully unprepared to launch a search for the physical manifestations of faith. No class, no textbook, and no grand rounds I could remember had ever attempted to ascertain the physical properties or merits of belief in God.

And yet, while nothing about my medical training prepared me for this, my interactions with patients, their families, and with people in general led me to believe that my hypothesis was sound. The idea that humans are wired for God, that we are custom-made to engage in and exercise beliefs, and that spiritual beliefs are the most powerful of that sort, felt like a truth that had always existed inside of me and inside of humankind to which I had suddenly gained conscious access. Like synesthesia, which we talked about earlier in the book, it was as if a physical process had risen to the surface, so that for the first time I was attuned to a primal human motive and a timeless source of physiologic strength and health.

Why do I suspect that belief in God is a primal motive or a survival instinct? Let me summarize the findings of this book that led up to my conclusion. We've examined how influential faith can be when cultivated by an individual, by someone caring for an individual, or by the relationship between the two. We've demonstrated that beliefs have physical repercussions, both positive as in remembered wellness and negative as in the nocebo effect. And we've explored how our culture, ethnicity, and daily experiences shape our beliefs and thus our physiology.

Then we delved deep into the workings of the brain, where we witnessed an astonishingly complex system in which patterns of nerve cell activation are created and stored, and in which life experiences mingle with genetics, constantly shifting the cellular pathways that determine all our thoughts, movements, feelings, and functions. We learned that people come into the world with hard-wired instincts (among others, fear of heights, or acrophobia, and fear of snakes, ophidiophobia), with the fight-or-flight response, and with the notion of being "whole"—of having arms, legs, and a torso. These are genetic predispositions. Our brains became wired with these strategies because they enabled the survival of our ancestors and the continuation of the species. We also unconsciously react to all the things that happen to us and to all our ideas with emotional markers, the logic and origins of which we have yet to understand.

The Burden of Mortality

B ut we haven't talked about the fact that humans are sad-
dled with an intelligence that threatens our very existence. While we are the most intelligent creatures on
the planet, outsmarting all other animals, we are also, ar-
guably, the only species that recognizes its own mortality, the
inevitability of death. In pondering such questions and facing
such facts, ignorance may be bliss because the recognition of
death can be such a torment, so depressing and anxiety-pro-
ducing in humans as to impair our survival. Because we are
the only species that can ask, "What will happen to me after I
die?," we must answer that question in a way that promotes
our survival.

Cicero is reported to have said, "All philosophy only talks
about one thing—death." I have come to believe that in order
to counter this fundamental angst, humans are also wired for
God. Whether or not God exists, our genes guarantee that we
will bear faith and that our bodies will be soothed by believing
in some antithesis to mortality and human frailty. So that we
will not be incapacitated by the acknowledgment and dread
of death, our brains harbor beliefs in a better, nobler meaning to life.

Karen Armstrong writes in *A History of God*, "Jews, Christians, and Muslims have developed remarkably similar ideas
of God, which also resemble other contemplations of the Absolute. When people try to find an ultimate meaning and
value in human life, their minds seem to go in a certain direction. They have not been coerced to do this; it is something
that seems natural to humanity." Belief in God is, indeed, natural to humanity, as natural as are our instincts to flee or
fight. As we saw earlier in the book, these predetermined instincts often result in common archetypes being developed,
our common fears and tendencies becoming the legends of
very different lands and peoples. Similarly, we develop ideas
of the almighty because it appears we are programmed "to go
in a certain direction."

After my shaving insight, I spent two years reviewing the religious and secular literature of the world for a common formula that would elicit the relaxation response. I found that in every nation, in every religion, the results were the same. Every culture had religious or secular practices that consisted of two basic steps—a repetitive focus and a passive attitude toward intrusive thoughts. There was transforming power in prayer, no matter what the words, from a Hindu prayer to the Catholic "Hail, Mary, full of grace," from Judaism to Buddhism, Christianity, and Islam. There were multitudes of descriptions of the peaceful state these religious practices elicited. Furthermore, I found many examples of secular approaches that brought forth the physiologic relaxation I'd seen in practitioners of Transcendental Meditation. These were scientifically proven techniques such as Lamaze breathing, autogenic training, and progressive muscle relaxation exercises.

Life Significance

Whether or not you believe in God *per se,* you attach purpose and significance to your life. Of course, individuals choose to manifest this wiring, this preset instruction, in very different ways. But we all derive the most intense strength and solace from seemingly transcendent qualities of life.

Some people look to children for their inspiration because children are untainted and ripe with possibilities. For others, gardens are deeply soothing, a profusion of color and life, constantly reborn. At their best, music and art can inspire generation after generation of listeners and admirers, as can natural wonders—mountains mingling with clouds, ocean tides never ceasing, and a sun that emerges every morning having been swallowed by the horizon the night before.

Faith in God, however, seems to be particularly influential in healing because "God," by all definitions of which I am aware, is boundless and limitless. It is part of our nature to believe in an almighty power lest our health be undermined by the ultimate and dreadful fact—that we may succumb to illness and that all of us must die.

I describe "God" with a capital "G" in this book but nevertheless hope readers will understand I am referring to all the deities of the Judeo-Christian, Buddhist, Muslim, and Hindu traditions, to gods and goddesses, as well as to all the spirits worshipped and beloved by humans all over the world and throughout history. In my scientific observations, I have learned that no matter what name you give the Infinite Absolute you worship, no matter what theology you ascribe to, the results of believing in God are the same.

Furthermore, I fear that the language in this chapter and in others in which I've discussed the spiritual experience will seem strained and inadequate, no matter how carefully wrought. Humans have always known this frustration, trying to represent that which is mystical and divine in finite, limited terms. And by our very mind-sets—pigeonholing science and religion, mind and matter—most of us are uncomfortable linking God and genes, spirituality and nerve cells.

An Organic Craving

But despite the inadequacy of our vocabulary and philosophy, the craving for divinity is fully and organically articulated in us. Jack Miles, a former Jesuit priest and a member of the *Los Angeles Times* editorial board, wrote in his recent book *God: A Biography,* "His is the restless breathing we still hear in our sleep." And Gallup polls demonstrate that 95 percent of Americans say they believe in God. Of course, we don't know what form God takes for those who answered the questionnaire. But it's uncanny to think that nearly all the citizens of our country agree on the presence of an almighty being.

Scientists feel this hunger as keenly, if not more so, as does society at large. Polls tell us that the majority of scientists call themselves atheists. But there is an old saying: If a little science takes one away from God, a great deal of science brings one back to God. Physicists, in particular, find themselves in a primordial quandary. So precise are the vast number of variables they know must have converged to cause the Big Bang, so unlikely are the coincidences and so preposterous the timing of the episodes that gave birth to the universe billions of years ago, that they have to choose between thinking that all of life is a miracle or an outrageous fluke. Similarly, the emerging chaos theory suggests that even the seemingly haphazard, innumerable events of life—the ripples in a pond, the snap of a flag on a flagpole, tiny aberrations in heart rhythms—may indeed be predictable and measurable if studied long enough with sophisticated computer and mathematical models. Detecting designs and patterns where no designs and patterns were previously apparent can produce tremors of faith in even the most stalwart scientist.

Reviewing a host of new books linking science and religion, *Wall Street Journal* writer Jim Holt says, "As far as contemporary science can tell, nearly everything about the universe—its knack for self-organization; its fine-tuned potency to bring about galaxies, life, consciousness; its sheer existence—is vastly improbable. This would seem to suggest that we are here because of a deliberate supernatural design."

Evidence of Purpose: Scientists Discover the Creator, one of the books Holt reviewed, is edited by Sir John Templeton, known for his success in steering mutual funds. One of my mentors, Sir John has devoted a foundation and his energies to studying the scientific basis of God. I have served as a member of an advisory board of the John Templeton Foundation and have had the opportunity to meet and talk with Dr. Owen Gingerich of Harvard University, Dr. Daniel H. Osmond of the University of Toronto, and Dr. Robert John Russell of the Graduate Theological Union, all of whom contributed chapters to *Evidence of Purpose*.

These authors argue persuasively that so improbable are the chances of the elements combining as they did to create life as we know it, so appealing is the theory that a "deliberate supernatural design" is at work in our lives, there is evidence that the universe was thoughtfully, not randomly, designed. In his book *The Physics of Immortality: Modern Cosmology, God, and the Resurrection of the Dead,* cosmologist Frank J. Tipler also contends that it will eventually be possible for theology to be encompassed as a branch of physics, and for science to answer the question "Does an omnipresent, omniscient God exist?"

Nobel laureate and physicist Leon Lederman has facetiously named one fundamental and stubbornly evasive factor "the God particle." The God particles—or Higgsons particles as they are better known, are like backboards off of which other primary particles of the universe bounce. A sequence gives the bouncing particles tangibility, or what we call mass. Without Higgsons, particles would be massless spirits jetting around space at the speed of light, no particle heavier than the next. Scientists believe that Higgsons are responsible for launching what we call "creation," in which myriads of matter and recognizable forms of life, the structures of the entire universe, were born. Many contemporary researchers hang their hats on the Higgson discovery, either presuming that particles spawned the miraculous happenstance we call "life" or that the Higgson was a pawn in a masterful, ethereal game plan. But I believe that no matter how eagerly scientists chip away at the mystery of our existence, the ultimate mystery of our origins and of the origins of this remarkable universe will remain impenetrable.

The Ultimate Mystery

Author Kathryn Harrison put it this way: "The modern world's replacement of faith with science means that, for most of us, there is no Mystery, only mysteries, and that . . . we are about to solve [those]." Our society subjects everything to empirical analysis, trying to reduce the unknowns and eventually to contain the whole world in neat statistical columns and formulas. Then perhaps we can make the wildest variables such as destiny, human choices, interpersonal relationships, and all other mysteries succinct and predictable.

Even when we acquire new information, even when we conquer mysteries, we feel vaguely empty and unfulfilled. And faith is the only long-term solace. In part that is because faith in an Infinite Absolute is the only adequate counterforce to the ultimate facts of disease and death.

But it is also because faith permits an appreciation for the unseen and unproved, generating a kind of hope inaccessible by reason. Ms. Armstrong writes that the earliest men and women worshipped gods "not simply because they wanted to propitiate powerful forces; these early faiths expressed the wonder and mystery that seem always to have been an essential part of the human experience of this beautiful yet terrifying world."

Transcendent Faith

I have found that faith quiets the mind like no other form of belief, short-circuiting the nonproductive reasoning that so often consumes our thoughts. Our bodies are very good at healing us but all too often we hinder this process, worrying that a cough could be indicative of something far worse because we've read or heard so many worst-case scenarios in the media, doubting that we have the strength to overcome it without help because that's what a host of advertising agencies and pharmaceutical companies have told us. These worries and doubts bring on the fight-or-flight response with all of its stress-related symptoms and diseases and blunt our evolutionarily honed healing capacities. Perpetual worries and doubts also make an impression on our nerve cells so that the body too frequently "remembers" illness and health threats in the nocebo effect phenomenon we've discussed.

But because faith seems to transcend experience and base reality, it is supremely good at quieting distress and generating hope and expectancy. With hope and expectancy comes remembered wellness—the neurosignature messages of healing that mobilize the body's resources and reactions.

Barbara Dawson's "Miracle"

I believe this is what occurred in my patient Barbara Dawson's case. Four years ago, Ms. Dawson told her surgeon, "God hasn't failed me yet," as she refused the operation he recommended for the cancer raging in her throat. Looking only fifty of her seventy-one years, Ms. Dawson said she'd rather die than have half her jaw and some of her teeth removed to extract the tumor.

Two daughters stood by her that day, as she weighed her options to battle the cancer, metastatic squamous cell carcinoma. The daughters betrayed none of their fears nor the trepidations being felt by her other five children. Having watched their mother survive the death of their father when they were still young, raise and send them to college on a teacher's salary, and overcome several heart attacks, heart failure, and the problems of chronic diabetes, they wanted to believe what she believed—that God would save her.

"But Ms. Dawson, the tumor could grow out to here," the head and neck surgeon said, gesturing to show how it might bulge and distort her face.

"Well, if it does, I'll knit a hat for it," she quipped. Ms. Dawson didn't feel she needed the operation; she was certain that a less aggressive approach with radiation therapy would work. But she couldn't have been prepared for how devastating the following months would be. She was hospitalized for weeks as radiation treatments deadened her taste buds, salivary glands, and the roof of her mouth. Swallowing proved next to impossible, and she suffered from both malnourishment and dehydration. Her heart problems recurred because often the heart medications she tried to swallow came out of her nose instead.

And yet at the time of this writing, five years have passed and Ms. Dawson has not had to knit a hat for her tumor. The throat cancer has disappeared. She has kept off the seventy pounds she lost during the course of her illness, beating a weight problem that had dogged her for years. Ms. Dawson also has a new companion, her first love affair in nearly twenty-five years. Her internist and surgeon call her a medical miracle—a term physicians have used more than once to account for her recoveries.

Eschewing surgery any number of specialists would have said was necessary for her survival, Ms. Dawson fought cancer with treatments she believed in: radiation therapy, a standard cancer treatment for decades, and another powerful method that has existed since the beginning of time but has often been disregarded by the medical community. She unflinchingly believed in her treatment decisions, in her medicine and caregivers, and in God's power to heal her, if it was His will.

No matter how frail and vulnerable she looked to those of us who cared about her, Ms. Dawson was a powerhouse of faith. It was as if every cell in her body functioned with the conviction that God had more for her to accomplish in life. She prayed daily, as did a prayer chain of family and friends that stretched across the country. "My kids pray for my health," she explains. "I pray for a pure heart. I pray to be a loving, healing person."

Later in the book, we'll talk more about the important point Ms. Dawson makes, that even though we have tremendous healing resources to call forth, a focus on health is unhealthy. This was something Ms. Dawson had always understood about prayer, having learned to pray while attending a black Pentecostal church as a child. Her minister there professed the merits of having a "secret closet within himself" to which he would retreat for an hour of prayer every day. That is why she called me to her bedside twelve years ago when she heard me teaching her hospital roommate a mental focusing technique to elicit the relaxation response. Because of her religious background, Ms. Dawson accepted wholeheartedly the idea that she could use the relaxation response to reap significant, long-term health benefits. She elicited the response faithfully, spending twenty minutes once or twice each day in quiet meditation or prayer.

Over the course of the twelve years I've known her, Barbara Dawson has taught me extraordinary lessons. But is she a medical miracle? Yes and no. The word "miracle" is much more widely used by the general public than it is in medicine. Physicians use the word "miracle" very judiciously, believing as we do that there is little that science cannot explain or will not eventually be able to explain. And if you take into consideration the role of Ms. Dawson's faith, which I believe helped her beat the considerable odds she faced when she decided to forgo surgery, remembered wellness does scientifically explain her recovery and disqualify it from miracle status.

I think that lay people are drawn to the word "miracle"— despite the strict requirements that medicine, the Catholic church, and others have of the word—because they instinctively appreciate the movement of faith and remembered wellness in their bodies and in their lives.

But we now know from the data we've seen in previous chapters that faith moves in us, but not in necessarily mysterious ways. We are beginning to be able to explain the way that physiologic mechanisms transmit and materialize faith to produce healing. This leaves us to ponder the truly remarkable fact that our brains/bodies are so equipped. And rather than thinking that science debunks miracles, I choose to believe that science underscores the awesome, and perhaps even miraculous, design of the human body.

I believe that all of us have the wiring that predisposes us to find faith enormously healing. But few of us are conditioned to respond to a diagnosis in the way that Barbara Dawson did. We let the illness define us. In our often harried search for relief from pain and suffering, we often miss what we are really looking for, and what our bodies really crave. Self-esteem is a good example. Gloria Steinem has called self-esteem "a revolution from within"—realizing that the cause of women's rights she has championed is often undermined because women and men lack the confidence required to learn from one another and to share their political and personal power. She suggests, and I agree, that if citizens and leaders of nations were more confident, the world would be less competitive and more cooperative, less aggressive and more peace-seeking.

However, self-esteem is not enough when it comes to struggling against illness. When a woman discovers a lump in her breast, when a man experiences chest pain, when people are jolted by symptoms they associate with serious illness, their images of themselves as strong, vigorous, and healthy are often instantly dampened or destroyed. Throughout life we see others succumb to freak or violent accidents, to sudden or prolonged illnesses, always dreading—either consciously or unconsciously—that we are next. Panic and fear, with their accompanying arousal of the fight-or-flight response, take colossal bites out of self-esteem, no matter how hard we try to master their influences. The brain also stocks its shelves with memories of everything you've ever heard about cancer, with all the random details of heart attacks and other diseases, so that to believe in yourself, you have to defeat not only your own fears but those passed on to you over a lifetime of learning.

Supreme Healing

No matter how caring the health care providers, no matter how positive and confident the outlook of the patient, the naming of an illness and even the idea of "recovering" from "sickness" instill new and usually negative messages in the brain. Although we want to believe that we can empower our bodies to do anything, we are burdened with a new definition of ourselves as "sick" and "weak," with their associated pathways of nerve cell firing and communication dictating physiologic responses. Unconsciously or subconsciously, we harbor what can become self-fulfilling prophecies—that our luck has run out, that we are prone to illness, that we have brought disease upon ourselves, that medicine can't cure everything, that doctors paint rosier pictures than may be merited, or that disability, loss of independence, suffering, or death are imminent.

That's why I have come to believe that faith in a bigger, stronger force is so influential. Faith in the medical treatment, faith in the health care provider, and faith in the relationship forged between you and your healer are wonderfully therapeutic, successful in treating 60 to 90 percent of the most common medical problems. But if you so believe, faith in an invincible and infallible force carries even more healing power. For believers' physical health, it is a supremely potent belief.

That's why I argue that our genetic blueprint has made believing in an Infinite Absolute part of our nature. By the process of natural selection, mutating genes deemed faith important enough to the survival of our forefathers and mothers that we were endowed with the same tendencies. Ironically then, it can be argued that evolution favors religion, causing our brains to generate the impulses we need to carry on— faith, hope, and love becoming part of the neuromatrix with which we approach living.

A Visceral Soul

Outlining the functions of the brain, Dr. Damasio writes, "The truly embodied mind that I envision, however, does not relinquish its most refined levels of operation, those constituting its soul and spirit. From my perspective, it is just that soul and spirit, with all their dignity and human scale, are now complex and unique states of an organism." Taking this view, the mind and body are indivisible, our beliefs and emotions have physical origins and manifestations, and the soul—previously considered elusive and ephemeral—is remarkably involved in the visceral as well.

With our visceral soul intact, belief in God lends us a will to live we would not have without God. This is, of course, why religion becomes more important to us as we age, a trend noted by historians and supported by the recent surge in interest in spirituality among baby boomers who are now reaching middle age. Perhaps this urgency to find God is also born of the coming end to the millennium, which, similar to the deaths around birthdays we examined earlier, could be a deadline or a lifeline for many people who are anticipating the year 2000.

As we draw closer to the inevitable facts of declining health and death, the torment grows and our need to venerate our current experience expands proportionately. As Samuel Johnson said, "When a man knows he is to be hanged in a fortnight, it concentrates his mind wonderfully." This is why people in the midst of life-threatening diseases find solace in religion, why congregations pray for those who are hospitalized, and why some Catholics want priests to read final rites for them. This is why people struggling with AIDS, often those whose lifestyles have been condemned by mainstream religion, so often embrace spirituality to live their remaining days, overcoming whatever barriers might keep them from believing in God or in practicing faith. Nothing makes God more real to people than the prospect of death. But whether we recognize it or not, death is an ever-pressing reality for a brain that wants to overcome obstacles, for an organism guided by one dominant principle—to keep you alive.

Ms. Armstrong writes that her "study of religion has revealed that human beings are spiritual animals. Indeed, there is a case for arguing that *Homo Sapiens* is also *Homo religiosus*. Men and women started to worship gods as soon as they became recognizably human."

Individual Pointlessness

Without infusing life with meaning, Dr. Susan Blackmore, senior lecturer in psychology at the University of the West of England, writes in her book *Dying to Live: Near-Death Experiences*, humans are left to ponder "our individual pointlessness." Because pondering pointlessness can have devastating effects on our health, it appears safe to speculate that our brains evolved to crave meaning instead. What a concept. Even if you are a proclaimed atheist or agnostic, your brain hungers and is soothed by the idea of purposefulness. Our brains do what must be done so that we will "be fruitful and multiply," and our genes are a kind of evangelist, our biology constantly promoting in us the power of faith.

Thus, some contend that humans invented the idea of God over time as a crutch or balm to stave off an otherwise cruel reality. In this vein, Dr. Blackmore writes:

> The problem with evolution is, and has always been, that it leaves little room either for a grand purpose to life or for an individual soul . . . the idea that God created us for a special purpose is a lot more palatable than the idea that we just got here through the whims of "Chance and Necessity," as the French biologist Jacques Monod put it, even though it has no evidence to support it and provides no help in understanding the nature of the living world. And people will fight, and even die, for the ideas they like best.

She continues:

> This idea [of meaninglessness] can be just too horrible to accept and we will go to enormous lengths to invent something more substantial to hang on to. "If I see through this there must be something more!" or "Now I understand the creation of illusion, I can see the 'real' thing." I believe that all these attempts are missing the scary truth: that there is nothing substantial to hold on to—not even oneself.

In this interpretation, evolution has engendered self-deception en masse. If death is the period to the sentence of life, perhaps the evolved brain has played with the punctuation, trying to escape the inevitable. Even scientists looking for a God particle, for some sense of the material world, may deceive themselves. So says physicist Edward Kolb of Fermi National Accelerator Laboratory: "The easiest thing in science is to find what you are looking for."

Implanted by God?

A nd yet, others maintain that the capacity for faith and for conjuring God—what many would call the soul—was implanted by a Maker who wanted us to know Him, Her, or It. Do we have faith because God intended us to worship, pray, yearn, and be fulfilled by believing in an Infinite Absolute? And if so, when in the course of evolution might God have intended the soul to be manifest? Are lesser forms of life influenced by human beliefs? You'll recall the ways in which I tried to quantify this with Lady Raeburn and data, which I could not replicate, that suggest that animals and plants may be affected by beliefs. Obviously this is a matter of dispute about which far more research needs to be done.

Which Came First?

I believe that this is a proverbial chicken-or-egg question, and that it will be impossible for science to say which came first—the animal or the soul, man or the concept of God, a life in which faith became a survival strategy or the genes that made life and faith possible. Despite science's unceasing attempts to quiet it, the Mystery of our existence reverberates.

But my scientific journey has led me to what I believe is a more important point, at least for my purposes as a physician. It does not matter which came first—God or the belief in God. The data I have presented is that affirmative beliefs and hopes are very therapeutic, and that faith in God, in particular, has many positive effects on health.

In what I know must seem coldly analytical to those who fervently believe in God, faith is a win-win situation when it comes to our bodies. Believing that God exists, or simply believing that God is food for a brain that craves it, allows humans to reap rewards in both improved health and in greater personal fulfillment. Faith is good for us, whether you believe that God planted these genes within us or whether you believe that humans created the idea of God to nourish a body yearning to survive, an artifice that made the prospect of all the days on earth more palatable.

If humans are indeed wired for God, and benefit from spirituality in the same important ways that every generation past and every generation to come will, how are we to incorporate this new fact of physiology? How will medicine, society, and individuals themselves adjust to this new consciousness of the unconscious predispositions that shape our everyday experience? Obviously, theologians, spiritual leaders, and individuals themselves must wrestle with the facts this research has revealed and with its implications. But in the pages and chapters that remain, I will address the medical and public health questions that center on remembered wellness and the faith factor.

Specific Theologies

I can say that, according to my investigations, it does not matter which God you worship, nor which theology you adopt as your own. Spiritual life, in general, is very healthy. However, I do think that the insights scientists have unveiled thus far about the workings of the brain, and the experiences my patients have had with the relaxation response, can lend us a few insights into how to worship.

As much as we desire to experience some imparting of the divine in Western society, we often deny the validity of highly intuitive encounters and of emotion itself. Emotion, you'll remember, decides for the brain and the body the value of information being processed, playing a far more important role in human physiology and mental function than Western society gives it credit for. And although we don't understand all the ways in which emotion works in our brains, the synesthesia expert Dr. Cytowic suggests that all of us know more than we think we know, that all of us are comprised of more primal instincts than we consciously recognize. We often do not allow for the inherent wisdom of the mind and the body to emerge, perhaps because we don't know how to access such wisdom or because we're conditioned to act on problems rather than to wait for answers to present themselves.

We know that mental focusing techniques that elicit the relaxation response quiet the mind and the body to a more substantial degree and with greater speed than any other means. We know that the experience seems to clean the slate of the mind, making it more receptive and creative. And we know that the experience feels very spiritual to some people, and that spirituality agrees with them, producing better health.

So perhaps there is something particularly powerful about intuitive or nonintellectual experiences of God or spirituality, the kind accessed in mental focusing, meditation, or prayer that incorporates the repetitive focus. In Western society we prefer that anything important to us be based on fact, empirically verifiable evidence, and rational thought rather than on intuition or belief. We have traditionally been very uncomfortable with the word "mysticism" and with "mysteries." Scientific researchers such as myself issue questionnaire after questionnaire, and make measurement after measurement, trying to precisely characterize the spiritual experience by its mix of mind/body influences, by the impact of human beliefs and a physical wiring that ensures that humans have spiritual beliefs.

Many mainstream religious denominations also walk a kind of narrow theological balance beam, invoking and enjoying the presence of God while associating passionate or transcendent spiritual experiences with cults, extremists, and hippies. Rather than enjoying the idea of a transcendent and relatively unknowable God—a being that defies exact description but nevertheless feels close to us, is good for us and for humanity—we are zealous in our attempts to pin personal, identifiable traits on God.

Trying to Know God

Armstrong says that a central motif of Judaism, Christianity, and Islam is the idea of "confrontation or a personal meeting between God and humanity" in which "God relates to human beings by means of a dialogue rather than silent contemplation." She is adamant that the overly personalized God, the God we insist must talk to us in the way that humans talk rather than in more enigmatic ways, "can become a grave liability." She writes, "He can be a mere idol carved in our own image, a projection of our limited needs, fears, and desires. We can assume that he loves what we love and hates what we hate, endorsing our prejudices instead of compelling us to transcend them. When he seems to fail to prevent a catastrophe or seems even to desire a tragedy, he can seem callous and cruel. . . . The very fact that, as a person, God has a gender is also limiting. . . ."

History is awash with the blood of religious wars. And whatever gains in public health we attribute to faith could be countered with the fact that a professed faith in God has so often been used to justify genocide and slaughter. Armstrong proposes that the overpersonalization of God, our fervent attempts to make the unknowable knowable, is to blame. Not only does it justify evil human aims, it saps religious faith of its energy, an energy we know has profound physical implications. She suggests that the intuitive or more mystical experience of God—common to all religions, peoples, and times—could transport religion and humankind, if only mysticism didn't seem to confine its effects to very disciplined students of meditation. And she cautions that perhaps people need mentors and leaders to guide their mystical quests for God.

Obviously, my research, and that of my colleagues, speaks to her concerns. Monks, rabbis, priests, and other disciplined students of prayer and meditation are not biologically different from you and me; they may pray in such a way as to evoke the spiritual and physical experiences our bodies are wired to exhibit. The relaxation response is likely to summon these experiences when one's beliefs are captured in the faith factor. But some of my patients report a kind of spiritual enlightenment the first time they evoke the relaxation response. And after just a month of eliciting the relaxation response, our research subjects demonstrated a significant increase in spirituality.

Religious leaders should be the ones to address the matters of controlling and managing spirituality. As far as medical science can tell, there are few if any dangers to the relaxation response and its prayerful applications. Instead, there are considerable health benefits to short periods of regular, unsupervised prayer or meditation that elicits the relaxation response. But it is disconcerting for some religious believers to think that everyone, with or without traditional religious affiliation or training, has access to the presence of a spirit that can be called God. They argue, if everyone has access to God in the comfort of their own homes by way of the relaxation response, who will need to belong to churches or temples? And without the structure of organized religion to steady the "divinely intoxicated" person, how will society control the actions of fanatics and extremists who claim communication with God fuels their deeds?

There is something to be said for the careful and reasonable guidance of elders and teachers when meditation and mental focusing techniques are practiced over long periods of time and under the intense conditions my colleagues and I have witnessed in retreats and monasteries. Otherwise, as I've said, strange or dramatic experiences are rare while general waves of peacefulness and tranquillity—strong enough that people believe they must be divinely imparted—are fairly prevalent. And society will continue to grapple as it always has with fanatics and extremists who invoke God's name to commit unscrupulous crimes.

The larger religious community will have to look to its leaders for clues as to how to digest scientific findings that, on the surface, may appear to threaten current religious beliefs or practices. My experience has been that most clergypeople embrace the methods of eliciting the relaxation response, for their own personal fulfillment and spiritual edification as well as for that of their parishioners.

Spirituality Heals

T he fact that we all share the potential to feel the presence of an external energy force, a God if you will, could be such a tremendously healing and unifying revelation for a diverse, strife-torn world. Many of my patients tell me that their belief-based elicitation of the relaxation response has broadened their religious views, made them more respectful of the spiritual quality of life, no matter what religion expresses it. It is as if the elicitation puts them in tune with other people, as well as with a spiritual presence.

But the idea that God is a product of beliefs, which are nonetheless critical to the species' survival, is startling to some people. Even though God is ultimately unknowable and unprovable, and can only be envisioned, conjured, and believed in by way of the faculties of our minds and bodies, it is hard for many believers to attribute their faith simply to their faith.

But, as disconcerting as the news may be for some, my medical pursuits maintain that it really makes no difference where this capacity for spirituality came from, from God or from some evolutionary mandate, only that it is ultimately very good for health and for humanity. It is a win-win situation to believe in an Infinite Absolute.

A bumper sticker says to "Expect Miracles!" We've seen that there may be physiologic reasons that the recoveries and cures we've often called miracles occur. And we've seen that mystical and spiritual experiences, which some people deem miraculous, are in fact possible and accessible by eliciting the relaxation response, although dramatic effects such as those we associate with miracles are rare.

So the adage "Let go and let God" comes closer to describing my philosophy when it comes to remembered wellness and the faith factor. To summon the healing effects of the relaxation response, you need to surrender everyday worries and tensions. People can call upon God or their particular object of faith to experience a succor unmatched by any other form of belief. When you let yourself focus, and get your harried mind out of the way of your body's natural healing ability, calling on the beliefs that mean the most to you in life, a peace that defies description may be possible.

I believe that the evidence is clear. As was true in Barbara Dawson's case and for all of us, our systems enjoy the results of our wiring, faith coursing through us with tremendous influence. With a visceral, inseparable soul and a genetic predisposition to soothe ourselves, we can better cope with the daily strain of life, and more fully appreciate the great Mystery of it all. Faith affirms life, perpetually and timelessly.

CHAPTER 10

OPTIMAL MEDICINE, OPTIMAL HEALTH

When the Oklahoma City federal building was bombed in 1995, assistant fire chief Jon Hansen became a familiar face to most of us as he gave reporters the daily increasing numbers of confirmed dead his rescuers had unearthed in the rubble. But even though no survivors were found any later than the second day after the explosion, Hansen was always careful to say that the rescuers had not given up hope.

As days and then weeks plodded by, victims were memorialized, suspects arrested, and the national psyche resigned itself to the fact that no place could now be considered safe and that fear and caution must dominate our thoughts now more than ever. But all that time, Hansen's team had to continue with their grim task, withstanding the odor and vivid images of death all around them, often with the teetering instability of the wreckage endangering their lives as well.

But it wasn't until the very end of their operation, when the bombed structure so imperiled the workers that they let demolition teams take over, that Hansen acknowledged the futility of hope. Before that point, he always maintained that the men and women working at the site could not continue without hope.

Just as hope gave the Oklahoma rescuers the strength to endure and allowed them to make sense of their participation in such a vile and senseless tragedy, humans, as I argued in the last chapter, have always needed faith to survive and to overcome the grim reality of mortality. Our convictions, the way we perceive and make sense of the world, are inevitable reactions to life and death. Religious faith is a particularly soothing form, but beliefs of all kinds assume tremendous influence over the body. And as we've seen, faith and hope do possess considerable influence over us, and they are made physically manifest in a phenomenon called remembered wellness.

But as naturally as faith and remembered wellness occur in us, they will not come as naturally to a medical system that has denied their validity. In this chapter, I'll focus on reintroducing belief-fostered healing into Western medicine. I'll present the enormous cost savings that I believe can be achieved by appreciating these mind/body influences, and which have already been realized in test programs around the nation. I also hope to guide you and policy-makers in considering how medicine can make practical changes, using remembered wellness across the board and reserving medications and procedures for those instances when they're needed and can be effective. Finally, I'll talk about the influence of unconventional medicine and the ways in which I believe it should be used.

The Medical Model: A Three-Legged Stool

I have proposed that the medicine of the future be like a three-legged stool, balanced and supported by these three components: self-care, medications, and procedures (see Figure 1). And this is the model on which my colleagues and I base our work at the Mind/Body Medical Institute.

The Mind/Body Medical Institute is perhaps the oldest of an emerging number of centers around the country trying to incorporate information about, and therapies drawing upon, mind/body interactions as part of mainstream medicine. In ten-week group meetings, my colleagues treat hundreds of patients each year, emphasizing the value of self-care, the things that individuals can do for themselves such as eating healthily, exercising, eliciting the relaxation response, and managing stress. We offer general healthy lifestyle programs and programs targeted to people who are living with cancer, AIDS, heart problems, chronic pain, infertility, menopause, and insomnia. We also make available to people many of the resources we use at the Deaconess Hospital—relaxation response tapes, books, and other materials that get people started in self-care regimens. (A list of the tapes appears at the end of this book.)

But we are also dedicated to training the trainers. Every

year, we teach hundreds of health professionals from throughout the United States and the world. We train clergypeople, educators, and corporate wellness personnel in the principles in this book, and we help them help their patients, congregants, students, and workers learn the self-care techniques that can be beneficial to health. Also, under the program direction of Marilyn Wilcher, we have established affiliates of the Mind/Body Medical Institute around the country. Satellite programs at the following hospitals have taken up our approach: Mercy Hospital and Medical Center in Chicago, Illinois; Morristown Memorial Hospital in Morristown, New Jersey; Memorial Hospital Southwest, Memorial Health Care System in Houston, Texas; Riverside Methodist Hospital in Columbus, Ohio; Baptist Hospital in Nashville, Tennessee; and St. Peter's Medical Center in New Brunswick, New Jersey.

There are, of course, other mind/body programs in conventional and unconventional medical settings around the country introducing Americans and the health care system to the healing our beliefs and behaviors can bring. But I think the strength of the Mind/Body Medical Institute and its affiliates is our commitment to teaching and to an integrated approach, drawing appropriately on all the assets of the three-legged stool. We do not dismiss the potential of individuals to heal themselves, nor do we recommend the use of conventional medicine or unconventional medicine to the exclusion of the other. But we do emphasize the cost-effectiveness and scientific merits of self-care and the need to reduce our reliance on medications and procedures that cannot help us, no matter who dispenses them.

The Economic Incentives

So there are already some programs in place that are changing the way that medicine is being practiced. But what will it take for dramatic and widespread change to occur in health care? To a large extent, the answer is economic incentives. An economic boon, mind/body approaches could, by a conservative estimate, save the system over $50 billion per year in wasted health care expenditures.

My colleagues and I have ample evidence not only that mind/body approaches are an inexpensive and largely untapped resource, but that actively engaging in them reduces cost and improves quality of care. In 1991, principal investigator Dr. Margaret A. Caudill, other researchers, and I collaborated on a study of the effects of mind/body medicine on patients with chronic pain, a population that you may remember from studies mentioned earlier tends to overuse the medical system, trying to gain relief from pain. Dr. Caudill's highly successful approach is described in her groundbreaking book *Managing Pain Before It Manages You.*

Dr. Caudill's team introduced 109 HMO patients to the relaxation response, exercise, nutrition, and stress management in weekly meetings that lasted for ten weeks. She found that after one year there was a 36 percent reduction in clinic visits among these patients—an estimated net savings of $12,000. In the second year, the savings were $24,000. And in a 1990 study, in which Dr. Caroline J.C. Hellman served as principal investigator, my fellow researchers and I achieved a 50 percent reduction in office visits, this time at another HMO, Harvard Community Health Plan, and with primary care patients.

Similarly, in a twenty-year study of patients in one of the country's largest HMOs, Kaiser Permanente, the authors concluded that the failure of the health care profession to acknowledge and address psychosocial concerns—stresses that produce symptoms not yet measurable by Western science— has the potential to bankrupt the health care system. Dr. Nicholas A. Cummings and Dr. Gary R. VandenBos learned that the system becomes overloaded precisely because 60 to 90 percent of doctor office visits are from patients manifesting physical symptoms of emotional distress. They write:

> Patients with concerns and symptoms related to societal, interpersonal and work difficulties do not tend to receive appropriate and responsive care within general health care systems. A perfunctory and un-

sympathetic response is most typical. . . . If the patient, however unconsciously, translates this distress
into a low back pain, the patient is immediately "re-
warded" by the physician in the form of X-rays, laboratory tests, medications, and return visits.

This can, the authors go on to say, encourage the patient,
either sub- or unconsciously, to continue having the pain, to
fulfill the expectation. This is the nocebo effect, the opposite
of remembered wellness.

Engendering Unrealistic Expectations

You'll recall the study in which people with chronic pain
who thought of themselves as disabled experienced
more pain and disability. Often the system encourages
patients to develop or maintain physical symptoms to achieve
credibility. Patients also learn to return to doctors and overuse
the system because health care professionals make them feel
as if being completely pain-free is the goal. And patients return because they do not get the compassion and attention
they desire the first time, or because they're pursuing diagnostic proof of a mystery pain or problem that may not yet be
measurable.

In the case of stress-related complaints, Kaiser Permanente's answer was to make mental health services widely
available, a solution that proved highly cost-efficient. Eighty-
five percent of the patients they studied benefited from brief
episodes with mental health professionals who obviously
cared about the patients and helped them arrive at proactive
solutions to their problems.

Mental health counseling is helpful to many people, particularly if worries or problems are complicated or of long standing. But there are many patients, such as Jimmy Burke, who
you'll recall endured almost continuous anxiety attacks, who
may not benefit from counseling alone. Psychiatry is sometimes as reductionistic as so much of medicine, failing to ap-

preciate the cumulative nature of stress-related illness, or the fact that a constellation of negative thoughts, doubts, and worries can directly contribute to medical problems.

Closely examining the 567 medical complaints patients presented in their medical clinics, Dr. Kurt Kroenke of Bethesda, Maryland's, Uniformed Services University of Health Sciences and Dr. A. David Mangelsdorff of Fort Sam Houston, Texas's, Brooke Army Medical Center found that 74 percent had no identifiable organic cause, and that in two-thirds of the cases, patients went on to receive diagnostic evaluations, which cost, on average, between $110 and $409 per patient. These tests revealed an organic cause only 16 percent of the time. And the cost of pursuing an "organic diagnosis" was high, especially for complaints such as headaches ($7,778) and back pain ($7,263), both of which are common to people experiencing stress. Only 55 percent of the patients received treatment in the end and often the treatment was ineffective.

I've often noted that 60 to 90 percent of physician office visits are related to mind/body and stress-induced conditions. But to arrive at the billions per year in cost savings, I settled on 75 percent as an average. I estimated from our data that half of doctor office visits—or 37.5 percent—could be eliminated with a greater emphasis on mind/body health and remembered wellness. Using 1994 statistics, there were approximately 670,000 practicing physicians in the United States who reported an average of 74.2 patient visits per doctor per week, for a total of 3,858.4 office visits per doctor that year. Each visit for an established patient cost an average of $56.2. Thus, the average cost per year was 670,000 x 3,858.4 x $56.2 = $145.3 billion. By reducing these visits by 37.5 percent, the cost savings would be $54.5 billion dollars, for one year alone.

This does not include the savings incurred by the decreased use of drugs, both prescription and over-the-counter versions, the decreased use of laboratory tests, and the decreased use of procedures. And if the effects of unconventional medicine are largely those of remembered wellness, as I will contend, and we reduce the reliance of Americans on unconventional medicine—on which at least $13.7 billion dollars is spent each year—we can achieve billions of additional cost savings.

A New Strategy

I believe that in 60 to 90 percent of doctors' visits, remembered wellness and other self-care techniques can be the treatment of choice. In more acute or chronic situations, these techniques can enhance the success of drugs, radiation, or surgical approaches. And by appreciating patients' beliefs and values, medicine can return to patients the dignity and sense of control that too many patients say is missing from their encounters with physicians and health care facilities. The medical profession needs to devise a better strategy to treat the vast majority of patients—three-fourths of the people who come in for medical office visits. In these cases, it's unusual for our current diagnostic techniques to consider the source of the problem, and our pharmacologic and surgical treatments are highly ineffective.

Looking at this same issue from another perspective, Dr. David Sobel revealed in a 1993 article in *Mental Medicine Update* that 25 percent of physician office visits are for problems that patients could treat themselves. If patients were empowered and better equipped to diagnose and treat themselves, as they now do 70 to 90 percent of the time with the average aches and discomforts they experience, a fourth of doctor office visits could be affected. In other words, a healthy percentage of the 25 percent of patients who make unneeded and costly demands on the health care system could be taught to treat themselves.

Dr. Sobel summarizes that when mind/body medicine is incorporated into standard medical practice, when patients are encouraged to play an active role in their health care and maintenance, the total number of outpatient visits decreases by 17 percent, visits for minor illnesses go down by 35 percent, and hospital surgical ward stays can be reduced by 1.5 days. Office visits for acute asthma problems decrease by 49 percent, visits by arthritis patients decrease by 40 percent, and visits for acute pediatric illness decrease by 25 percent. In childbirth, which carries with it enormous costs, cesarean sections can be reduced by 56 percent and the need for epidural anesthesia during labor and delivery is reduced by a staggering 85 percent.

Mind/body approaches can be very cost-efficient, encouraging independence and discouraging an overreliance on the medical system. When doctors rely more on the things that patients can do for themselves, they order fewer tests, fewer procedures, and fewer medicines, all of which reduces costs dramatically.

But when is it appropriate to rely on self-care? And how can a person know which legs of the three-legged stool need to be applied to a medical problem at any given time? The answer to the first question is straightforward. Self-care, including remembered wellness, should become a habit. Again, in this book, I'm focusing on belief-engendered medicine but it's optimal to pursue health with good nutrition, exercise, stress management, as well as other good habits. It should be part of your daily routine so that you do your best to prevent mind/body medical conditions from developing. If and when illness does develop, no matter what the illness, self-care and remembered wellness can have positive effects. In other words, self-care and remembered wellness should be used to treat virtually every disease or illness.

And yet, in this book, we've covered a plethora of medical conditions in which belief plays a major role—either positively in remembered wellness or negatively in the nocebo effect. While this list is by no means complete, here are the conditions demonstrated to be affected by belief in the studies cited in this book:

- Angina pectoris
- Bronchial asthma
- Herpes simplex (cold sores)
- Duodenal ulcers
- All forms of pain—backaches, headaches, abdominal pain, muscle pain, joint aches, postoperative pain, and neck, leg, and arm pain
- Fatigue

- Dizziness
- Impotency
- Weight loss
- Cough
- Constipation
- Congestive heart failure
- Nausea and vomiting during pregnancy
- Rheumatoid arthritis
- Postoperative swelling
- Hypertension
- Diabetes mellitus
- Degeneration of heart muscle
- Drowsiness
- Nervousness
- Insomnia
- Skin reactions to poisonous plants
- False pregnancy
- Deafness
- Death (clearly a major nocebo effect!)

Of course, these symptoms and diseases can be caused or influenced by many factors other than your beliefs. The point I'm making is that in many cases the disorder may have some origins in the mind/body realm and the treatment falls into the realm of self-care. Remembered wellness and other forms of healthy living can make a tremendous contribution to healing these maladies.

But what about the other two legs of the three-legged stool? I want to be perfectly clear that pharmaceuticals and procedures can, without the aid of remembered wellness, cure or heal people in the circumstances in which they're needed. It would be foolhardy and dangerous not to use them in these circumstances. Disregarding them would be denying yourself the incredible, proven scientific treatments that have given humans the ability to overcome disease and live longer and better-quality lives.

Many medical texts would be required to document all the specific circumstances to which I am referring. But to give you an idea of the treatments that are of essential and undeniable benefit to us, when properly used, I've developed the following list (which is by no means inclusive):

- Immunizations for polio, diphtheria, smallpox, whooping cough, measles, hepatitis, and tetanus
- Anesthesia for surgery
- Surgery for trauma injuries
- Dentistry for cavities and prostheses
- Antibiotics for bacterial infections
- Cataract removal and lens replacement to prevent and cure blindness
- Hearing aids for hearing loss
- Vitamins for diseases caused by vitamin deficiencies
- Hormone replacement therapy for diseases caused by hormone deficiencies
- Prosthetic limbs for amputees and the disabled
- Joint replacements for damaged joints
- Drugs for congestive heart failure, cardiac arrhythmias, lymphomas, mood disorders, and schizophrenia
- Pain-alleviating drugs for acute pain and for some kinds of chronic pain
- Artificial heart valves for obstruction or incompetence of heart valves
- Cardiac pacemakers for heart rhythm disturbances
- Cardiac defibrillators for heart cessation
- Blood and plasma transfusion for blood and plasma loss
- Organ transplants for livers, hearts, kidneys, and lungs

While I am a strong proponent of self-care, I firmly recommend that you make an initial visit to your doctor at the onset of a recurrent or dramatic symptom. It's vitally important to rule out the existence of a medical problem that requires the invaluable resources of scientific medicine. And as you become more attuned to your body's average aches and pains, you'll learn when doctors' visits are appropriate. The reduced office visits and the cost savings I associate with the implementation of remembered wellness do not demand that patients eschew seeing their doctors. On the contrary, I hope that incorporating mind/body medicine into medical practice will mean that patients have more satisfying interactions with doctors, in which doctors appreciate the many ways the body can exhibit pain or duress, encourage patients to care for themselves, and instill appropriate expectations for patients of what medicine can do for them.

As we have seen, mind/body interactions may actually cause many conditions, making the impact of remembered wellness particularly curative. And likewise, diseases and illnesses that owe their development to a number of biological and environmental factors, many beyond the realm of mind/body interactions, cannot be successfully treated with remembered wellness alone.

The Emerging Good News About Self-Care

There is evidence emerging, however, that self-care can be very influential in even the most unexpected circumstances. Dr. Michael H. Antoni and his colleagues at the University of Miami conducted an intriguing study of healthy gay men who had not previously been tested for the AIDS virus, or HIV. Randomly divided into two groups, all the men were tested for the HIV antibody. One group met weekly and received self-care training in the time leading up to their receiving the test results; the other received none of this training. The men in the first group learned progressive muscle relaxation, assertiveness skills, and other stress management techniques, and also discussed "cognitive restructuring," in which people can break their habits of automatically thinking negative thoughts and instead introduce affirming, remembered-wellness-inducing thoughts.

Seventy-two hours before and one week after the men were notified of their results, they gave blood and answered questionnaires about their emotional and mental states at the time. In the end, the men who tested positive for the AIDS virus and who had received self-care training showed no significant increases in depression, in contrast to the men in the control group who tested positive. Correspondingly, the blood tests revealed that the men in the self-care group who tested positive had significantly higher counts of helper-inducer and natural killer cells—immunological allies on which the body relies to fight disease. In this study, Dr. Antoni and colleagues suggest that relaxation techniques and a willingness to adhere to the protocol buffered both the psyche and the immune system from the potential harm of the diagnosis.

Another study, conducted by Dr. Fawzy I. Fawzy of the UCLA School of Medicine and colleagues from UCLA and other institutions, demonstrated the value of self-care in the potentially life-threatening cases of malignant melanoma. Patients who received education on the disease itself, on basic nutrition, on stress management and coping skills, and who received psychological support in a group setting and one-on-one with staff members, were less apt to have the disease recur and less apt to die than patients who didn't get this help.

It's becoming increasingly clear that the way in which we perceive ourselves, and the way that we cope with daily life, can impact the way that cells interact in our bodies. But rather than engage in simplistic, dangerous either/or thinking and disregard the marvelous life-saving and life-enhancing merits of the pharmaceutical products and technical innovations we're afforded today, we need a balanced approach. We need all three legs of that three-legged stool.

The Moderate Approach

Yogi Berra is alleged to have said, "If you come to a fork in the road, take it." I couldn't agree more. To many, a fork may represent a divergence of paths. To me, the fork represents the joining of two roads—traditional and mind/body medicine, in the balanced approach I advocate. I've enjoyed the middle ground in my career, trying to apply science to realms considered unscientific. I've been conservative in studying what many consider progressive subject matter, trying to remain dispassionate and objective about beliefs—which are often passionate and highly subjective. And I've felt compelled to make my medical findings accessible to mainstream people, by publishing books and by teaching and lecturing in nonmedical settings, and to remain at Harvard Medical School where I could continue to establish my work in the scientific community.

I digress for a moment to acknowledge the former Dean of the Faculty of Medicine at Harvard Medical School, Dr. Robert H. Ebert, who was unflinching in his support of my earliest inquiries into Transcendental Meditation and mind/body connections. While others criticized my work for being beyond the pale, Dr. Ebert maintained, "If Harvard can't take a chance, who can?" He is now chairman of the board of trustees at the Mind/Body Medical Institute.

Over twenty years ago, when I wrote the popular book *The Relaxation Response*, some elder colleagues told me that direct communication with the public was unacceptable behavior at Harvard Medical School. Since that time, I have generally found that academicians and physicians who are successful at translating and marketing their message to the public leave academia and "go public." There are many reasons for this, not the least of which is the difficulty of straddling two disparate worlds—one that loves sound bites, another that demands measured, precise pronouncements; one that begs for the big picture, another that isolates and reduces illness to its basic components.

But I have found this fork very gratifying. Of course it has meant that my work is not easily categorized. Proponents of unconventional medicine don't know if I'm friend or foe, journalists get exasperated by my demands not to be pigeon-holed, and some of the old guard of medicine have not always known what to do with my findings about the relaxation response or self-care. But I believe this fork, this combination of roads, better represents the human condition than arbitrary niches, and it has made my work attractive and helpful to large numbers of patients. Patients suffering from high blood pressure who might never have subscribed to meditation, considering it cultish, elicit the relaxation response because its results have been scientifically reviewed and published. And longtime practitioners of yoga or meditation techniques have appreciated the scientific credibility made possible by these same results. Both religious people and nonreligious people, liberal and conservative thinkers, can find merit in self-care and in the prospect that beliefs, as diverse as they can be, have medicinal value.

My preference for the balanced approach and the middle ground brings me to points I want to make about Western society's recent surge of interest in unconventional medicine.

Unconventional Medicine

Many people are turning to unconventional medicine because of the weaknesses they attribute to the conventional system. They like that less traditional healers acknowledge the existence of medical problems that cannot necessarily be measured in scientific terms, as well as the powerful movement of an energy or force that Western medicine cannot verify. They also may be drawn to herbs they believe are more natural or to procedures that seem less invasive. And while I've acknowledged how much medicine needs to change to empower patients and take advantage of patients' faith and beliefs, I dispute the wisdom of turning from one set of drugs and procedures to another set of drugs and procedures. The most "natural" form of healing is that which the patient does for him or herself. Too often it seems that patients are switching their loyalties and their reliance from one set of solutions to another, each of them inadequate in their own way, instead of bolstering their own internal healing.

This is why I do not like to use the term "alternative." I do not believe patients should use unconventional therapies to the exclusion of traditional medicine or medical advice. I prefer the term "unconventional," which, in my mind, describes methods that are not "mainstream" and do not, at this point in time, meet the aforementioned standards of scientific credibility—measurability, predictability, and reproducibility. Thirty years ago, mental focusing and meditative techniques were considered "unconventional," but with my findings and those of others about the physical state brought forth by specific means, they became part of the mainstream. In fact, a recent Gallup survey reveals their prevalence, indicating that 26 percent of the U.S. population practices meditative or relaxation techniques.

Is Remembered Wellness Unconventional?

Bㅤut given these definitions, which camp does remembered wellness fall in—conventional or unconventional? It's hard to say whether or not the phenomenon known as the placebo effect is mainstream. It has undoubtedly existed as long as humans have, and it is always at work in medical interactions, whether or not doctors and patients acknowledge its effects. But it is not emphasized in medical textbooks or lectures, it is not yet a part of the automatic thinking doctors bring to the bedside, nor are patients necessarily being encouraged to learn about it or use it. So I would have to say that right now remembered wellness is still unconventional even though it has more proven scientific merit than other therapies in the unconventional realm, such as bee pollen and shark cartilage.

Just as I said was true of *much* of traditional medicine, I believe that all of unconventional medicine, until proven differently, should be considered to be effective by means of remembered wellness. Nevertheless, for many people, remembered wellness as evoked by unconventional medicine is very successful.

Obviously, since I have written an entire book heralding remembered wellness, I do not intend to demean unconventional practices by saying that all the cures they produce come from within patients themselves. But while traditional medicine can boast of some breathtaking, scientifically verifiable cures and remedies, unconventional medicine cannot yet do so. Nevertheless, remembered wellness as fostered by unconventional medicine can work very well.

A Conspiracy Theory?

Some advocates of unconventional medicine entertain a conspiracy theory, that pharmaceutical companies, research hospitals, and physicians have combined forces to keep new, and often less expensive, remedies from being tested and introduced into practice. And although I've offered examples in which I was dissuaded from studying unorthodox methods, I do not believe that conspirators exist. Although there are disincentives in the system that should be eliminated, I also know that many scientists do what I have done: quietly test and try to quantify the claims of unconventional healers. The majority of them would not be afraid to bring a seemingly far-out idea to the forefront if they had enough test results to prove its worth.

Furthermore, in the medical circumstances I presented earlier, the effectiveness of traditional treatments was almost always immediately recognizable. Not only was the success of a treatment almost immediately apparent but the success was pervasive, helping nearly all of the patients affected most of the time. Many unconventional treatments have been around for a very long time, but their positive effects, if present and above and beyond those of remembered wellness, are still questionable. Acupuncture is a case in point. If its inherent healing effects were equivalent to those of proven scientific remedies, they would already have been recognized by Western scientific medicine.

The National Institutes of Health has established the Office of Alternative Medicine to investigate the healing properties of unconventional medical practices so that perhaps someday we will be able to acknowledge success that is not brought about by remembered wellness. But for now, we should appreciate the menu of healthy options we enjoy, using our positive beliefs to empower all curative methods.

I urge you to talk to your doctor before you begin a regimen of unconventional treatments. Or, if you know your doctor will not approve or handle this discussion well, find a doctor who is more open-minded. My former student Dr. David M. Eisenberg of Beth Israel Hospital in Boston found that 72 percent of patients who pursue unconventional medicine do not tell their physicians about these pursuits. And before the relaxation response became widely known in the medical establishment, my patients often complained that other doctors did not acknowledge the role that self-care habits played in improving blood pressure or overall health results. But increasingly it will be common for conventional and unconventional health practitioners to coordinate patient care, to exchange information and track a patient's progress together.

Weighing the Risks of Unconventional Medicine

When considering unconventional treatments, and when talking to your doctor about them, apply the same risk-benefit analysis to unconventional therapies as you would to conventional therapies. Ask yourself, "Do the benefits of the therapy exceed its risks?," "What relief can I expect from the treatment and is it worth the money?," and "What could go wrong, either by using this technique or by ignoring another option?" And just as I'll recommend that you do with traditional medicine, trust your instincts and don't submit to a treatment you don't believe in. Don't try acupuncture if you're scared of needles. Or conversely, if ancient Chinese medicine fascinates you, study it and pursue it with care.

The prevailing risk in unconventional medicine is the cost of treatment that, like conventional medicine, can be significant, except that in many cases, unconventional treatments are not covered by insurance or included among benefits in HMOs or other health care plans. Again, Americans spend an estimated $13.7 billion on unconventional approaches every year. Because this money will probably come out of your own pocket, you'll want to consider all the ways in which remembered wellness can be activated, and the gamut of health benefits that can be garnered from self-care, before you pay someone else to elicit healing that is already within your grasp.

Generally speaking, there is very little risk of physical harm from unconventional medicine. In homeopathy, for example, patients are treated with what is, essentially, water that previously contained an allegedly active substance. As long as treatments are not uncomfortable or unsanitary, acupuncture, chiropractic, and massage therapies are relatively safe. You'll want to check on the sanitary preparation and storage of herbs as well, and make sure you are not allergic to them.

But I believe the biggest risks in using unconventional medicine are of overlooking a serious medical condition, ignoring cures or better treatments that traditional medicine has to offer, and adverse interactions between conventional and unconventional therapies. An herb can react poorly when combined with a prescription drug. But again, these risks can be averted if you maintain good communication with your physician, and if the physician and unconventional healer communicate as well.

The Use of Placebos and Informed Consent

I believe that the kind reassurances doctors offer go a long way toward helping patients. This is all that's needed to engender remembered wellness. I do not propose the use of placebos in this avenue of healing. Doctors and caregivers should not lie to patients about their conditions nor deceive patients about the medicinal value of drugs or procedures we offer them. Because our society is so conditioned to expect that we will receive tangible medicines from doctors, it would be very difficult for us to go "cold turkey" and stop using medications immediately and completely, even for the conditions over which these drugs have little inherent healing effect. We doctors can, however, gradually reduce medications as patients become self-care practitioners and regain their identities as healthy people.

I expect we will continue to be a society that demands informed consent, even if the risks that get explained to us may cause us harm. It would be best for caregivers and patients alike if our society was less litigious so that kind reassurances could prevail over frightening warnings in medical offices. But caregivers should keep in mind that, with our knowledge of the nocebo effect, informed consent documents can be hazardous in and of themselves, and that we should introduce risks and statistics to patients only in a context of warmth, confidence, honesty, and concern.

The Time Is Right

Having spent decades verifying mind/body connections, I believe the time is finally right and that Western medicine is moving, albeit more slowly than the public would prefer, toward profound change. I truly believe that our paths are converging, that despite perpetuating Descartes' fallacy, health care professionals desire the same meaningful relationships that patients want. This is what the future holds, according to December 1994's *Economist*, in which Dr. Thomas Inui, Harvard's professor of ambulatory care and prevention and head of the Department of Preventive Medicine and Ambulatory Care, says that he believes the days of doctors serving as "mere diagnosticians, and as prescribers of sophisticated drugs, are numbered." He predicts those jobs will increasingly be the domain of technicians, robots, and other machines, "whereas doctors will be sought for their counsel and social wisdom, returning to their roots as healers."

With these new definitions, however, will come new responsibilities. As we'll see in the next chapter, the doctor-patient relationship must change. Patients and doctors need to learn to let beliefs work. With a more balanced approach, taking faith and remembered wellness into account far more often, we can aspire to a higher form of medicine. Dr. Inui relates to this, remembering how, as a young physician serving a Native American population, he was asked by a Najavo in New Mexico what he did. Never knowing quite what to say, Dr. Inui replied, "I give out pills." "Ah," the questioner said, "you are the low sort of medicine man. We have two sorts. The high sort, we go to for counseling and care."

CHAPTER 11

TRUST YOUR INSTINCTS, TRUST YOUR DOCTOR

S everal years ago, the Mind/Body Medical Institute established an affiliate at the Riverside Methodist Hospital in Ohio. One of the physicians who greeted me at the opening ceremonies of this satellite center was Dr. Donald J. Vincent, currently director emeritus of gerontology. Dr. Vincent was quick to share a tale in which the placebo figured prominently in his tenure as a country doctor.

Beginning in 1939, Dr. Vincent worked for seven years as the sole physician to 1,500 people who lived in rural Utica, Ohio. He took over the medical practice and office of a Dr. Kass, who died after serving as the town's doctor for many years. Dr. Vincent began settling into the office by cleaning out the pill room—a room or closet common to offices of country doctors, who often dispensed pills and pharmaceutical items themselves. He noticed a tall jar of coated, purple capsules labeled "placebo" on a shelf. "I took one look at the jar," Dr. Vincent recalls, "and, having gone to medical school and having completed a year of training in internal medicine, I considered myself a scientist, so I marched out the back door and dropped it into the waste can. And I felt very pristine about doing so."

But as his medical practice got underway in Utica, Dr. Vincent was surprised that a significant number of patients with a variety of medical conditions complained that his treatments were not working as well as had Dr. Kass's. One lady who suffered from osteoarthritis said, "The prescription you gave me didn't work as well as those purple pills Dr. Kass gave me." A man who struggled with hypertension inquired, "Might you have the purple pills Dr. Kass used to give me for my blood pressure?" It wasn't long before Dr. Vincent got on the phone to the drug company that produced the purple pills to order a gallon jug. And because his patients believed in them, the placebos worked wonders.

Dr. Vincent says he learned more about medicine in his seven years as a country doctor than during any other time in his nearly sixty years of medical practice and teaching, and the truths he gleaned from those experiences are still fully applicable in spite of all the advances medicine has incorporated since then. It wasn't just the purple pills that made Dr. Kass's treatments work, Dr. Vincent learned. "There's no question that having to humble myself enough to use the purple pills made me a better doctor. In those days, I had a few things to learn about listening to and paying attention to patients. It's really the purpose of the person giving the purple pills that affects patients," he explains.

An Interest in Humanity

The young Dr. Vincent, armed with the latest information science had to offer, relayed his "purpose" to patients on their visits to his office. But within a matter of months, Dr. Vincent found that his patients prized his listening and attentiveness even more than his mastery of the latest discoveries, even more than the dictates of his prescription pad. And long after he moved and began practicing in a city medical center, he received calls and visits from patients from Utica, sometimes from elderly widows who wanted advice or reassurance, sometimes on matters entirely unrelated to medicine, like the sale of real estate. If Dr. Vincent couldn't help them, he put them in contact with someone who could.

It's not hard to figure out the "purpose" or intent that, over time, Dr. Vincent exhibited and embodied. Very simply, he cared about his patients. He did more than care *for* them, more than evaluate their health status and prescribe treatment. He cared *about* them. Really good physicians exude such care and warmth. They learn to recognize how desperately a patient like Mrs. Johnson, whose weekly bridge game is a mainstay in her life, fears losing her eyesight, which would make her unable to play cards. Or how hard it is for Mr. Miller to take an hour off for a checkup, due to fierce pressures at the mill where he works. Or how Bobby Casey's back pain acts up every track season, each time his coach predicts he'll break his brother's legendary record in the 100-yard dash.

As I've pointed out throughout this book, these values and beliefs not only imbue physical life with meaning, they affect and influence physical health. Your thoughts and feelings about the daily experiences of your life both originate from and transmit signals to your body, neurologically and biochemically instructing and changing your health. The stress a man feels when a birthday nears, by which time he feels he should have more to show for himself, can contribute to his death. The expectation that a spinal tap will result in a headache can bring on the headache.

Since the majority of the medical complaints that bring Americans to their doctors' offices are stress-related and it's clear that self-care approaches such as the elicitation of the relaxation response have considerable success in battling stress, doctors and patients need to learn to affect health with positive outlooks and remembered wellness. We've seen that faith is a health-affirming player in human life. Our wiring disposes us to desire and be soothed by life's meaning. And as our understanding of the brain expands, the mounting evidence reveals an organism that inseparably tangles body, mind, and soul.

So in this chapter, I'll suggest ways in which you can enjoy the benefits of remembered wellness within the status quo medical system, to improve doctor-patient relationships, to draw upon these relationships to chart the best course of treatment, and to take advantage of belief in standard or unconventional medicine. Although my primary focus is on improving conventional medicine, the truisms offered here can easily be applied to maximizing your relationships with healers and unconventional medical practitioners as well.

There are, as I've said before, three modes of engaging remembered wellness. This mechanism for self-healing, a kind of in-house pharmacy, is summoned by your beliefs, by your caregiver's beliefs, or by the beliefs generated in your partnership.

How can you ensure that you're getting medical care that takes mind/body influences into account and believes in the power of the individual to do something about these medical problems? There are no easy answers to this question. Today, health maintenance organizations and other insurers hold most of the cards in the health care game, not only telling doctors how many patients they must see each day but limiting a patient's choice of doctors. And just when you find a good doctor, your employer may switch HMOs or insurance plans and force you to look for another "preferred provider." What's worse, an estimated 43.4 million Americans do not have *any* health insurance, cannot develop a partnership with a physician, and live in fear of illness necessitating care. But whenever possible, I urge you to trust your most precious commodity—your health—to someone who signals to you that your spirit and outlook are important considerations.

Your search for the right caregiver may also be complicated by the fact that, as I said earlier in the book, many doctors today remain committed to the traditional view, relying heavily on drugs and procedures, and neglecting the healing assets of self-care. But I've developed a few guidelines that may help you make the most of your options. And frankly, these steps can help doctors and patients alike to mobilize remembered wellness: 1) Identify the other's important beliefs and motivations; 2) Talk about and be willing to act on beliefs; and 3) Let go and believe.

I'm directing my attention to improving the traditional doctor-patient relationship but it's wise to apply these rules to your interactions with unconventional medical caregivers as well. It's important for you to get a sense of your doctor's basic beliefs and motivations. You want a caring doctor who is open to your being an active participant in your care, who believes in the power of belief as well as the power of medications and surgery. You want someone who not only cares *for* you, but cares *about* you.

1. Identify the other's important beliefs and motivations.

Before choosing a doctor, ask friends, colleagues, nurses, and pharmacists for recommendations. Find a physician who emanates friendliness and caring, who is cautious about prescribing medications and treatments, and who welcomes patient input and participation.

Since your health plan probably dictates which physician you can use, you may need to do some research before you choose a plan. Don't be afraid to call and ask the plan's representative how much time their internists or family practice physicians are allowed to spend with patients. Alan Raymond, author of *The HMO Health Care Companion: A Consumer's Guide to Managed Care Networks*, recommends you go one step further, asking doctors, "Is there anything about the way you are paid by the HMO that will affect your care of me?"

It's important to seek medical care in a setting that you believe will do you the most good. If you equate excellence with the high-tech offerings of a prestigious medical center or teaching hospital, you'll be better off getting your care there than would a person who is intimidated by a "big-name hospital" and who likes the convenience and informality of a local doctor's office or a community hospital. If antiseptic smells and institutional hallways scare you, you may prefer a facility that cultivates a comfortable, homelike atmosphere.

FIRST IMPRESSIONS

A recent Harvard University study reveals that our first impressions and instinctual reactions are usually on-target. According to a 1993 article in the *Journal of Personality and Social Psychology*, Harvard psychology professors Nalini Ambady and Robert Rosenthal showed undergraduate students thirty-second and shorter video clips of a variety of teachers in classroom settings. The sound was either turned off or scrambled in the film clips so that study participants were only evaluating teachers' body language or nonverbal behavior. The professors compared the study participants' immediate impressions during these very quick glimpses of teachers to end-of-semester evaluations submitted by students who had taken classes with the filmed teachers. Nearly three-quarters of the time, the intuitive reactions the study participants reported matched the reactions of students who had taken semester-long classes with them. Drs. Ambady and Rosenthal suggest that perhaps the human tendency to form impressions so quickly is evolutionary, that in order to thrive the species may have been forced to develop a keen sensibility for distinguishing friend from foe.

To harvest the fullest measure of remembered wellness, we have to trust our instincts. If you already have a doctor, give some thought to your interactions. Has the physician offered non-drug-related solutions to physical ailments and problems? Does the doctor seem interested in you, ask you about your work or your family? Do you feel you have his or her full attention? Has your doctor ever asked you what you thought was the source of a medical problem or symptom? Does your doctor make you feel good? If you're unsure what your doctor thinks about the power of belief, ask! Mention that you read this book and that you're interested in what he or she thinks about mind/body interactions.

This is what Dr. Vincent meant when he described "purpose." Your doctor doesn't have to share your particular religious or philosophic views. But to develop a trust that will manifest remembered wellness, you need a doctor who cares about the whole of you, who makes you feel that your life is more than a sum of body parts and processes. Dr. Francis Weld Peabody, the first director of Harvard's Thorndike Memorial Laboratory—the place where my research career began—wrote in his 1927 medical classic *The Care of the Patient:* "One of the essential qualities of the clinician is interest in humanity, for the secret of the care of the patient is in caring for the patient."

By and large, people who get admitted to medical schools have common attributes: a desire to help people and an aptitude for science. But over the course of four years of medical school, the time in which aspiring doctors are expected to become acquainted with and understand all the diseases and biologic functions of the human body, they get used to seeing symptoms and signs of illness and injury separate from actual patients. Furthermore, their knowledge of specifics is tested far more than their ability to assess overall patient well-being. Doctors often take these habits with them into medical practice, emphasizing specifics over wholeness, body over mind, leaving many patients feeling underwhelmed by their compassion or interest.

Of course it's possible that a less-than-attentive doctor may summon the first type of remembered wellness by recommending a treatment you happen to believe in, maybe because a friend of yours was helped by the treatment or because you read about the procedure in a magazine. It's possible that a doctor who emanates more confidence than caring can garner the second type of remembered wellness, that of the belief and expectations of the caregiver. But to harvest the most influence remembered wellness has to offer, you have to have faith in your doctor. You have to feel good about your doctor to develop this trust.

ADVICE FOR PHYSICIANS

In the same way I recommend patients find out their doctors' motivations, doctors need to look for their patients' beliefs and motivations, soliciting and listening to the way in which patients describe their health and the activities in life that matter the most to them. We need to be alert for the fears patients express, even in the shy, embarrassed way many patients relay fears. This is the art of medicine that often takes some time for a physician to learn; it's a much more intuitive process than the scientific assessments we spend the bulk of medical school and residency learning to make.

One of my patients experienced high readings every time his blood pressure was checked, a trend that started years ago when this man, who is of average weight, sat on an examination table in a doctor's office that collapsed underneath him. You'll also recall the story of the woman infatuated with her internist who only had high readings when *he* checked her blood pressure. When we doctors watch for and pick up on these individual characteristics, the subtleties and seemingly incidental details that make people unique, we make more appropriate medical judgments and activate remembered wellness, all at the same time.

2. Talk about and be willing to act on beliefs.

It's important for patients and physicians to talk about and be willing to act on beliefs. Earlier in the book you may recall a study in which patients who asked more questions experienced fewer medical problems. It concluded that patients should not just place health matters into trusted hands but take matters into their own hands as well. So let your doctor know about tensions or worries that could contribute to or exacerbate your medical condition. Trust your instincts, and trust the doctor who values your impressions and assessments.

Many patients feel cheated if they leave a doctor's office empty-handed, and doctors often cater to these expectations by offering prescriptions even when a patient's condition doesn't necessarily warrant it. This is a form of remembered wellness—giving you a pill that you expect to help. But in the process of doing this, doctors often underestimate a patient's willingness and motivation to try self-care, to change a diet, increase exercise, and pursue other drug-free therapies.

If you are a person who dislikes taking pills, who experiences side effects more dramatically than others, or who doesn't believe in medications for your condition, you're wise to communicate this to your doctor. Knowing your wishes, your doctor may be less hasty to prescribe a pill. If medication is the best or only course of treatment, the physician may prescribe a smaller dose or more closely monitor your experience with the drug. In any case, if the doctor is attuned to your stated preferences, you'll be more likely to adhere to treatment. And as we saw in the earliest chapters of the book, adherence or following a doctor's orders—even if the prescription is for a placebo—can prove life-saving in and of itself.

TRUST INSTINCTS

In everyday life, we often recognize gut instincts. We can tell when a waiter or waitress is overburdened and distracted. We get a sense of whether or not we're being taken seriously by the car mechanic. We can often tell when someone we're talking to glazes over and stops listening to what we're saying. But when it comes to the medical profession, we are often intimidated or scared by the subject matter and we disregard our true feelings and reactions, even though brain research tells us that emotions are critically important decision-makers in our minds/bodies.

You probably wouldn't put up with a hair stylist or barber who rushed through your haircut, who looked at his/her watch constantly, or who kept interrupting your appointment with less-than-important phone calls or conversations. You wouldn't trust a stockbroker who didn't return your calls promptly. You wouldn't enroll your child in a day-care facility in which the director plainly didn't listen to you or your child. Nor is it likely you would give your business to any professional who, unapologetically, made you wait forty-five minutes past a scheduled appointment.

TALK ABOUT PROBLEMS

The American Medical Association recently determined that patients wait an average of twenty minutes in their doctors' waiting rooms. This may be compounded by another fifteen- to thirty-minute wait in the examination room, this one less comfortable because the patient has changed into a breezy cloth or paper gown. These signals of neglect make patients angry, and more likely to sue. Malpractice suits are more often filed by patients who feel their doctors don't care, don't listen, are often late, or with whom it is difficult to schedule appointments.

Instead of getting angry, talk to your doctor about the matter. If that doesn't work, try to find another doctor. If you're routinely being asked to wait forty minutes to see your physician, or if you're enduring other poor manners or gestures that demonstrate a lack of concern, the faith you need to have in your doctor is being undermined and remembered wellness thwarted. Your body's amazing healing ability is the best friend you could possibly have in the world of medicine, and you shouldn't allow negative encounters with the medical profession to blunt this power.

HEALING WORDS

In George Bernard Shaw's 1911 play *The Doctor's Dilemma*, he describes the character Sir Ralph Bloomingfield Bonington in the following way: "cheering, reassuring, healing by the mere incompatibility of disease and anxiety by his welcome presence, even broken bones, it is said, have been known to unite at the sound of his voice." The sound of a doctor's voice, the words he or she chooses, the hope he or she can instill, and the time required to develop a good doctor-patient conversation promote health in ways many doctors and most insurers underestimate today.

In the June 15, 1995, *Patient Care* journal, Dr. Richard Letvak related a painful experience in which he believes his words engendered the nocebo effect in one of his patients. He wrote:

> I treated a backwoodsman who worked very hard— and worked alone—at logging. Twice, after cutting down a tremendous number of trees, he experienced shortness of breath, lightheadedness, and chest pain. Although he had no significant risk factors for angina, I suggested that he might be having heart pain and explained that we would see if medication made it better. That was his first and last visit to my office. He never filled the prescription. Instead, I later learned that my opinion had been so upsetting that he'd become depressed and abusive towards his wife.
>
> Eventually, the patient consulted a cardiologist. A stress test was ordered even though it didn't come close to simulating his usual everyday exertions. As might have been expected, the test confirmed that he could exercise at the maximum heart rate for his age without experiencing heart pain. Even if he had heart disease, symptoms would not be evident without extraordinary effort. The patient was offered a far more palatable explanation for his chest pain: He had probably overworked himself to exhaustion.

One truth in medicine is that diagnoses can't always be correct. The experience did, however, remind me to speak with care. There must have been indications that the patient was troubled by my assessment, but I didn't notice them. If I had sensed that I was going to provoke a crisis, I would have tried a more casual approach. After all, he didn't seem to be in immediate danger. I might have said that I wasn't sure what his problem was—it might be his heart or it might be nothing—and that we would see how he did over the next few months. But suggesting that the man might have a serious problem only made him feel worse.

Again, the quality of a conversation is crucial. Carefully chosen words can make an enormous difference to the patient who eagerly awaits a physician's conclusions. It isn't that doctors need to lie to patients. They just need to appreciate the import of their words, and of their power to evoke remembered wellness or the nocebo effect in patients. To offer optimal medicine, doctors need to have time to allay fears and to instill confidence and positive thinking. And insurers need to nurture the conversations that feed the doctor-patient partnerships that fuel remembered wellness and greater health.

3. Let go and believe.

Of the three rules I'm outlining, this is perhaps the most difficult for doctors, patients, and the health care system to adopt. We need to let belief work. As natural as it is for our bodies to heal us, it goes against our grain to let them do so. The prospect of "not doing something" is very threatening.

So we neglect the substantial therapeutic rewards of watchful waiting. The December 10, 1994, issue of *The Economist* credits Dr. Randolph Nesse, a psychiatrist at the University of Michigan in Ann Arbor, with being a leading theorist in a field called evolutionary medicine. Dr. Nesse believes that modern medicine may impair the "body's natural mending processes" by rushing in with our drugs and technologies. In this vein, "prolonged and watchful waiting" may be preferable to our societal expectation and medical norm—immediate intervention.

SURRENDERING CONTROL TO GAIN CONTROL

Immediate intervention makes patients and doctors feel "in control." And yet our desire for control is often excessive. We're conditioned to believe that our minds and bodies have to be at full-throttle most of the time. We think nervousness and the resulting adrenaline are good for performance, and that directed brain activity is the only productive kind. But in reality, a prolonged fight-or-flight response only hurts the body, and brain overload often decreases mental productivity. That is why I advise my patients not to focus on the results of eliciting the relaxation response. But the wonderful outcome is often that patients end up feeling more in control, and in more important ways than they did before.

Similarly I've found that doctors who surrender their excessive worry and perfectionism and who help patients draw upon mind/body assets are not only happier practicing medicine, they're more self-assured. And this assurance is readily communicated to patients in the doctor's demeanor.

The former country doctor, Dr. Vincent, says that using the placebo humbled him and made him admit, at least to himself, that he did not know it all and that he could not heal everything. This is a very uncomfortable admission for most doctors and caregivers, who, in their zeal to cure and heal, never want to be at a loss for an answer, never want to fail, never want to stop trying to make a sick person better.

One need look no further than the anesthesiologist whose mask was soaked with tears upon hearing his patient pray than to see that doctors, despite their apparent stubbornness, are still deeply moved by spirituality. It's sad to think that we have, as physicians and human beings, often closed ourselves off from our souls, from our basic instincts, and from abundant examples in our own lives and experiences in which we know that positive outlooks are influential and faith does enhance health. Distancing ourselves from beliefs, from the essence of human character, perhaps we think we can make "death" and "illness" less real, less painful. In our passion to control and banish illness and disease and to administer care as quickly and efficiently as insurers demand, we have neglected the scientifically proven and profoundly satisfying sources of hope for both our patients and ourselves.

Dr. Oliver Wendell Holmes's solution to this negligence was radical. He said, "If all drugs available were tossed into the ocean, all the better for mankind and all the worse for the fishes." I am not proposing tossing medicine overboard, but infusing our doctor-patient relationships with more common sense, reserving interventions of medication and procedures for conditions not alleviated by self-care, making the most of our internal assets and the most of our ingenious medical drugs and devices as I suggest in the three-legged stool analogy.

Our American penchant for problem-solving must now take into account the invisible but enduring contribution of remembered wellness, the internal, physiologic translation of the human spirit. We must make it part of the American mentality to appreciate the physicality of mentality, the momentum spurred by hopes and affirmations and not necessarily by the incarnations of American ingenuity, technologies, and medications. In the chapter that follows, I'll explore our societal conditioning and propose a healthier approach to the constant influx of news, often negative and worry-inspiring information, which can have so many troublesome side effects.

CHAPTER 12

THE ILLS OF INFORMATION

Pulitzer Prize–winning author Toni Morrison details the real danger of perceived danger in her book *Song of Solomon*. Morrison's characters, young Pilate and her brother Macon, spend weeks in dark, terrifying woods after their father is murdered, an experience that indelibly alters Pilate's life outlook. She says:

> Macon kept telling me that the things we was scared of wasn't real. What difference do it make if the thing you scared of is real or not? I remember doing laundry for a man and his wife once, down in Virginia. The husband came into the kitchen one afternoon shivering and saying did I have any coffee made. I asked him what was it that had grabbed hold of him, he looked so bad. He said he couldn't figure it out, but that he felt like he was about to fall off a cliff. Standing right there on that yellow and white and red linoleum, as level as a flatiron. He was holding on to the door first, then the chair, trying his best not to fall down. Then I remembered how it was being in those woods. I felt it all over again. So I told the man did he want me to hold on to him so that he couldn't fall? He looked at me with the most grateful look in the world . . . I walked around back of him and locked my fingers in front of his chest and held on to him. His heart was kicking under his vest like a mule in heat. But little by little it calmed down.

But then the man's wife comes into the laundry room and asks Pilate what she is doing. Pilate explains the predicament, releasing her hold on the man, "But soon's I let go he fell dead-weight to the floor. Smashed his glasses and everything. Fell right on his face . . . I don't know if the cliff was real or not, but it took him three minutes to fall down it."

"Was he dead?" Pilate's companion asks.

"Stone dead."

Morrison's portrayal of "death by belief" isn't a fictional fallacy. As we've seen in voodoo and in patients with a predilection for death, the nocebo effect is real, harmful, and potentially fatal. This is because fact and fiction are woven together in the human form, our thoughts and convictions about the world around us encoded in the physiologic world inside of us.

In *The Enchiridion,* the first-century Greek philosopher Epictetus wrote, "Men are disturbed not by things which happen, but by the opinions about the things." These opinions are formed over a lifetime of experiences and prioritized according to their emotional content by the brain's emotional engineering plant including the amygdala, the prefrontal lobes, and right cerebral cortex, and are physically represented by neurosignatures in our brains. We retain a stew of conscious and subconscious memories and impressions formed in life from our cultural upbringing, watching TV, reading, talking to friends, going to health clubs and drug stores, or visiting a friend in the hospital. All of these are ingredients in an internal milieu that the brain constantly assesses to prescribe appropriate bodily reactions.

The Side Effects of Information

I've devoted the first eleven chapters to enumerating the healing assets available to us because of the mind/body interplay. But the truth is, because so much of the information we feed our brains is pessimistic, violent, or anxiety-inspiring, and because our minds are trained to dwell on these aspects, our bodies also suffer the nasty side effects of nocebo, or negative beliefs. In this chapter, I'll explore the damage this onslaught of negativity can cause, and concentrate on the multitude of ways in which you, as an individual, can combat these effects. Our wiring ensures this is possible, but often we need to be reminded to rely on faith and internal healing. So I've included some tactics for you to remember wellness.

To remember everything but wellness, you need only take a

television clicker in hand for a minute or two. It isn't just that we spend hours watching explicit videos on MTV or that CNN regularly exposes us to the abominations of war. Americans also have a way of making even seemingly helpful, positive information stress-inducing. We allow information to manipulate us and to stir in us a multitude of unhealthy thoughts and feelings—inadequacy, guilt, shame, and futility, among others.

We harangue ourselves for not being perfect, for not living life with the panache portrayed in magazines or on TV. We adulate the firm-bodied, we exercise like zealots or wallow in guilt if we don't, choosing diet shakes over moderation, all of it designed to give biology less influence over our looks than hard work and self-denial. We aspire to parent perfectly, to juggle flawlessly the demands of work and home, and to have marriages and relationships of unwavering passion.

At odds with ourselves, convinced that we must overcome our natural tendencies rather than learn to enjoy and manage them, we are primed for sales pitches in which advertisers tell us how to fill the voids. Be it closet organizers, time management seminars, exercise equipment we use briefly and then banish to a closet or den, or a variety of pain relievers we're disposed to take at the first twinge of discomfort, our consumer habits are often based not on actual needs but on needs cultivated in us by advertisers.

In this climate, it's very hard to remember wellness. Remembering wellness requires a certain degree of self-confidence and affirmative inaction. Western society promotes outward self-improvement, not inward development. Our mind-set is to take *more* action, not less, to boost the body's abilities. We've grown up cherishing our "freedom of information" and admiring people who have "a thirst for knowledge," so our appetite for news about health and well-being is inexhaustible, our alertness to changes in our bodies sharpened with every report that tells us early detection is crucial.

Without necessarily attributing the division to Descartes, we've tried to steer our beliefs into a corner called private life, while in public we've conferred honor on empirical evidence, statistics, eyewitness accounts, and other so-called facts. We may let Disney movies and storybooks teach our children to "listen to their hearts," but we rarely encourage this inclination in adults, in diplomatic relations or in union negotiations, in corporate takeovers or major league sports, in politics or science, or in any of the news-makers in the modern world.

Exaggerated Threats

At the same time we underestimate the importance of faith and beliefs, we exaggerate threats to our health and well-being. We give illness more attention and more centrality in our society than it rightfully deserves. News is, by its nature, out of the ordinary or fresh, so the media doesn't promote our good health, the perpetual pumping of our hearts, the relatively smooth functioning of all our internal organs day after day, the operation of this inordinately complex machine that is so largely maintenance-free that we take it for granted. And often because the news media emphasize illness and disease, we assume a defensive and hyperaware position in health matters.

We also can't imagine anything worse than being seriously ill or disabled. We don't promote that the worst twist a life can take is hatred or abandoning one's morals. We dread disfigurement or disease far more. Advertisers abet this perception by making "pain-free life" the standard. And we've become so intolerant of illness that physicians are too quick to correct conditions best left unattended, too quick to order heart-bypass operations, hysterectomies, and other hasty, extreme solutions. We do all of this rather than instilling confidence in the body's ability to heal itself, or garnering hope—the key elements of remembered wellness. The medical profession's own fears of mortality and human frailty encourage a public disease with anything less than perfect health, making patients and families more likely to seek retribution in the courts if an outcome is undesirable.

In his book *Worried Sick: Our Troubled Quest for Wellness*, Dr.

Arthur J. Barsky of Harvard Medical School does not advocate mind/body solutions for our society's ailments. But he is forthright in condemning our propensity for exaggerating health threats, writing:

> We seem unable to enjoy our good health, to translate it into feelings of well-being and physical security. . . . We are pursuing perfect health and yet living all the while like invalids. We act as if perpetually poised on the brink of breakdown, while denying it at the same time. We don't live exuberantly but apprehensively, as if our bodies are dormant adversaries. . . .

He goes on to say, "We overlook the reality that most of us are healthy most of the time, the reality that the human organism has remarkable self-healing capacities for adaptation and survival."

The Roman philosopher and scholar Seneca said, "No man can have a peaceful life who thinks too much about lengthening it." And a wise Latin proverb asserts, "He who lives medically lives miserably." And yet Western society worships long life and physical beauty, not full, exuberant living or inner peace. Some cultures build restful siestas into afternoons, others consider family meals and dining their finest hours, still others gather for prayer or meditation at regular intervals throughout the day. If you ask Americans what good they did on any given day, you're likely to hear that they worked out, worked hard, did housework, yard work, volunteer work, or homework. The gauge of our goodness isn't based on who we are, but on what we do, not on the journey but on accomplishments, not on the quality of our relationships or perceptions but on the extent of our self-discipline.

This book, like others that advocate mind/body solutions and the power of positive thinking, can be used in the same workhorse, guilt-inspiring way. Perhaps you've added meditation or prayer to a vast to-do list, to the chores or requirements that you already feel badly about not doing regularly.

In this case, the good news of remembered wellness may be overwhelmed by the heart-pounding stress inspired by these obligations.

It's also very tempting to oversimplify this information, to become so impressed with mind/body connections that you attribute any decline in health to spiritual failure. Medical problems are, of course, the result of a number of variables including genetics and family history, environmental causes, personal history, health habits, and accidents. But because, as we've witnessed in our historical review, society often stigmatizes illness, mind/body medicine can, at its worst, be used to indict rather than empower people. And the last thing that people in the throes of illness need is to worry that they brought the condition upon themselves, or that a setback means that they lack the faith to heal themselves.

Nursing professor Barbara Lowery and her colleagues at the University of Pennsylvania found recently that 40 percent of the 234 breast cancer patients they polled believed that some personal behavior or personality trait had contributed to their getting the disease. An oversimplified reading of this book and others that encourage people to take full advantage of their healing resources could hurt patients, layering guilt on top of what is already a difficult emotional struggle. The danger of the mind/body message is that people will worry more, not less, about their conditions, and become convinced that negative thoughts will bring about a recurrence. I tell my patients that it's only natural to react with fear to a diagnosis of cancer or other disease, and to worry about what lies ahead. It's damaging, however, to let fear and worry become the focus of your life, and to let the label of illness say more about you than your personality and life experiences.

Many factors are involved in the development of disease and, particularly in the case of breast cancer, medicine does not know what causes the majority of cases, so blaming yourself is just plain erroneous. We have to be realistic about remembered wellness. It can help to the extent that any disease or condition is caused or exacerbated by mind/body interactions. If a disease progresses, despite the best efforts of self-care, it had a life of its own that was beyond the influence of remembered wellness. Sometimes the best medicines and the kindest, most renowned specialists cannot quell disease, and so it is with remembered wellness. Sometimes an uncontrollable biological entity prevails, despite our most fervent prayers, our most exuberant living, and our most hopeful attitude. Yet there should be no guilt involved. We do the best we can in difficult circumstances to preserve hope. That is all we can humanly expect from ourselves.

Health: A New Religion

Unfortunately, the American public has been conditioned to crave sound bites and simple messages. We avoid having to consider the complicated weighing of risks, or the multifactorial nature of our problems. We ignore steady, resilient, and good health and venerate an elusive and illusory perfect health. Dr. Marshall H. Becker of the University of Michigan wrote in a 1986 issue of *Public Health Reviews*, "Health promotion . . . is a new religion, in which we worship ourselves, attribute good health to our devoutness, and view illness as just punishment for those who have not yet seen the Way."

In yet another panacea for a species painfully cognizant of its own mortality, we often pursue health more than happiness, or confuse health with happiness. A 1982 survey of readers of *Psychology Today* found that 42 percent of the respondents thought about their health more than love, work, or finances. Forty-six percent said good health was the single most important source of happiness in their lives.

It's true that people who are highly introspective and self-conscious appraise their health as being worse than their less inward-looking peers. Indeed, we've seen that the act of looking outward in altruism or upward in religious life has healthy benefits. In his book *The Symptom Iceberg: A Study of Community Health*, D. R. Hannay uses community surveys of symptom reporting to show that the less active a person's religion, the more bodily symptoms he reports being bothered by.

I make a point of teaching medical students and young physicians the advice that His Holiness the Dalai Lama shared with me and my colleagues. The Dalai Lama was asked how to sustain the tranquil focus of meditation in one's everyday routine, outside of meditation. He answered, simply, "Focus on what is in front of you." It's not easy for any of us, clinicians or lay people, to live "mindfully," giving each moment and interaction our full attention as the Dalai Lama and some popular authors recommend, perhaps most notably among them Barbara DeAngelis in her book *Real Moments* and Dr. Jon Kabat-Zinn in *Full Catastrophe Living*. I struggle against my own tendency to entertain a thousand thoughts and worries simultaneously, to start a day with dread because my concerns and expectations weigh so heavily on my mind. But I've learned that when, for example, I am focused on my patients, I break my personal chain of thoughts and worries, which is essentially what occurs when you passively disregard everyday thoughts and mentally focus. When you focus on others, your mood will brighten. I believe this is the helper's high documented by Alan Luks and discussed earlier in the book.

I recognize how difficult this message can be for people who carry very heavy burdens such as serious illness, disability, or poverty. It is very hard for them to focus on the joy of the moment or on the people who need them. Often the way one views the scenery and people one encounters each day is utterly colored by these burdens.

Nevertheless, even in these cases, Dr. Barsky reminds us that paying attention to a symptom or problem amplifies it while distractions lessen our experience of it. Dr. Barsky believes this is why soldiers who are severely wounded can ignore their pain and continue fighting in the phenomenon known as "battlefield anesthesia." In battlefields and boardrooms, backyards and doctors' offices, the truth is that when you go on with your life, giving your full attention to each person and situation rather than allowing yourself to settle into a quagmire of burdens, your body is motivated to forget illness and pain, and to remember the strength and vitality associated with your full experience of life.

When you focus on health, however, "the mandate for self-discipline and self-control becomes so burdensome and so arduous that it begins to erode our sense of well-being and makes us feel increasingly insecure about [our] health," according to Dr. Barsky. This insecurity, this attention to our bodies, magnifies problems, sends inappropriate distress signals to the brain, and may contribute unnecessarily to fulfilling physical prophecies triggered by worry and fear.

The Nocebo Effect

The nocebo effect can manifest itself in many ways. As in remembered wellness, the body will attempt to abide by and demonstrate the suggestions the mind has been given.

Mass psychogenic illness (MPI) is a fancy term for a nocebo effect that occurs on a large scale. MPI is a common phenomenon in which groups of people—sometimes co-workers, schoolchildren, or others—develop medical symptoms and complaints as if stricken by an epidemic or exposed to an environmental hazard. MPI was responsible for the dancing manias found in Europe during the Middle Ages but its effects are also prevalent in modern times, although we might be inclined today to attribute them to "mass hysteria." Seven hundred people sought treatment in New Zealand in the 1970s for an exposure to fumes they believed, albeit incorrectly, were toxic. In the early 1980s, seventy-five Boston schoolchildren fell ill for no discernible reason during a grade school assembly. Factory workers have been sickened by bites from nonexistent insects. And recently, in the months following the terrorism in which sarin and other deadly poisonous gases were released in Japanese subways, passengers have taken ill on trains in which no gas was present.

In all these incidents, the belief in the existence of a disease-causing agent sparked a prevailing onset of symptoms. One nineteenth-century physician explained, "To become epidemic this disease must seize some popular idea or superstition, at once so *firmly* believed as to lay hold of the heart of the people, and so *generally* as to afford scope for the operation of pathological sympathy." Popular expectations can bring on these kinds of epidemics.

As is true of individuals who develop false pregnancies, or pseudocyesis, a potent belief can be the catalyst for authentic symptoms to appear despite the absence of a scientifically documented cause. In the New Zealand crisis, the impetus was a vile smell from a chemical spill off a damaged cargo ship. While authorities frantically tried to identify the contaminant, they ordered a major evacuation and prohibited travel in the supposedly poisoned area. Hundreds of people jammed hospital emergency rooms with symptoms of toxic inhalation from what was later found to be a smelly but harmless substance. A bad odor and some worried authorities caused a massive outbreak of the nocebo effect.

False memories can also be brought on with the suggestive power of nocebos. It's common for people to block out painful or traumatic memories and for psychiatrists, psychologists, or other counselors to help patients recall these significant experiences in the course of analysis. But sometimes, in overzealous attempts to unveil a source of anguish, counselors make the mistake of "suggesting" certain incidents to patients, or patients themselves develop accounts of events that they sincerely believe occurred. A belief-engendered memory can be a very dangerous thing, particularly when children mistakenly accuse their parents of physical or sexual abuse. My colleague Dr. Fred H. Frankel of Beth Israel Hospital in Boston recently wrote, "The desire to help the victims of childhood abuse heal is more than justified, but clinicians are urged to reflect also on the damage done by false accusations. Accepting the truth of long-forgotten memories elicited by therapy without corroboration can seriously injure and disrupt the lives of innocent people."

Richard Ofshe and Ethan Watters offer many accounts of false memories in their 1994 book, *Making Monsters.* In one account, a woman who sought advice from a counselor about a failing marriage was "cured" when she "revived" memories of participating in a Satanic cult that practiced ritual murders and cannibalism. It turned out that the woman had never had these horrendous cult experiences, so that, according to Mr. Ofshe and Mr. Watters, the patient ended up more confused and more traumatized by the "memories" suggested to her by the counselor than by the marriage problems she'd originally sought help to solve.

I believe that the nocebo effect is also at work in the recollection of past lives and in the much publicized claims of people who believe they have been visited by aliens. As in remembered wellness, these incidents are belief-generated but they are very real to those who experience them. And as was true in the cases in which physicians had difficulty distinguishing real pregnancy from pseudocyesis, beliefs can manifest themselves in impressive, convincing detail. Because our scientific understanding of beliefs and their repercussions is relatively new, doctors have much more to learn before we can properly isolate and recognize negative and manipulated manifestations of beliefs.

Knowledge Manipulated

In all these cases, knowledge was power. But knowledge did not always serve the public good as we expect it to. Information can be tricky because the more we know, the more we may be inclined to disregard our healthy beliefs and instincts. Take, for example, the phenomenon of medical student hypochondriasis. It's very common for young doctors, in the course of studying signs and causes of human illness and disease, to jump to conclusions that twinges of pain or other minor symptoms are signaling impending disease.

Edward Shorter of the University of Toronto reports in his book *Bedside Manners* that people of "higher social position," presumably those with greater access to medical care who enjoy better health than the poor, report a greater number of mild symptoms such as cuts, bruises, skin problems, and upper respiratory tract illnesses. In other words, people who do not have access to medicine do not have the luxury of focusing on minor ailments; they must confine their medical visits to emergencies. Elliot Friedson of New York University confirms this finding in *Profession of Medicine*, revealing that patients in poor, disease-ridden countries report fewer symptoms and fewer illnesses than Western physicians who examine them expect them to report. Obviously, as I noted in pain threshold studies, cultural differences can play a major role in determining one's outlook on health. However, it is striking that the healthier the society, the more attuned we are to minor health problems.

In February 1995, *GQ* reported on a survey showing college graduates and people who make more than $50,000 per year are least likely to be "very satisfied" with prescription pain medication. People at lower income levels, making $15,000 or less, and those who did not finish high school were more likely to be satisfied. Interestingly, "belief" in medical treatment seems to be undermined the better educated one is and the more money one makes, despite the fact that greater income generally affords people greater access to medical advice and care. The assumptions we make in society that education always improves our lot in life may not be entirely true in the case of remembered wellness. People who rely more on hopes and beliefs, who have learned to wait for healing, perhaps because they have no other option, may have an advantage over the information-obsessed.

Dr. Lowell S. Levin, professor at the Yale School of Public Health and one of the authors of the book *Medicine on Trial: The Appalling Story of Ineptitude, Malfeasance, Neglect and Arrogance*, said in an interview that women in particular are conditioned to consider all the stages of their lives "as disease states" for which they should seek medical attention. Five or six times more likely to use the medical system than men, Dr. Levin said in an interview, "Women are set up by the medical system to think that they are a danger to themselves, that every stage of their development is a pathology."

Dr. Levin believes in the "thirds" principle established by Dr. Philip R. Lee, assistant secretary of health in the Clinton administration. He explains Dr. Lee's theory that "one-third of medicine helps a great deal, one-third makes no difference, and one-third of it hurts us." Thus, he thinks that people play "Russian roulette" with a medical system that hurts them a third of the time. He insists, for example, that 90 percent of births could occur safely and less traumatically in the home.

In a medical profession still dominated by male doctors, Dr. Levin says, women are not taught to be self-protective. They're taught to trust the U.S. health care system, which, he says, treats their heart attack complaints less seriously than men's; produces inordinate numbers of false positives on Pap smears, high percentages of C-section births, and many more hysterectomies than are performed in other countries; promotes mammography despite its uncertain value; and has delayed yeast infection pharmaceuticals from becoming available over-the-counter.

Much of the health education and news with which we are bombarded is designed to heighten our worries, not soothe them. In particular, many drug companies both promote and play upon our tendencies toward hypochondria. In April 1994, *New York Times* reporter Elisabeth Rosenthal's article "Maybe You're Sick, Maybe We Can Help" pointed out that the consumers once told that the rumbling of acid indigestion could be well served by a two-cent dose of Alka-Seltzer are now being warned of a "serious medical condition" that necessitates a two-dollar-a-dose prescription remedy. Similarly, the article says, promotional materials distributed in doctors' offices inform people that what were traditionally "Excedrin headaches" may indeed be "migraines."

Dr. Marcus Reidenberg, editor of the journal *Clinical Pharmacology and Therapeutics*, believes that many drug companies "are taking symptoms of daily living, of normal existence, and converting these into diseases requiring medical treatment." He continues, "What the advertising does is to push patients to go to doctors when the symptoms are less severe than would normally cause them to make [appointments]."

Promotional campaigns emphasize symptoms and disease, rather than their products, the article suggests, because advertisers know "the more people obsess about an illness, the more likely they are to visit a doctor and the more prescription sales will rise." And the strategy appears to be successful. According to research by Scott-Levin Associates, a health care marketing organization in Pennsylvania, 78 percent of doctors surveyed said that their patients brought up symptoms they had seen raised in advertisements, compared to only 30 percent of doctors who reported this trend in 1989.

Breaking the Cycle

Our addiction to information often undermines or dooms the transforming power of remembered wellness. Recently, Corinne Kyle, a collaborator of mine on a study conducted by the famous polling company George H. Gallup International Institute, where she is director of research, was compiling some results and found a gentle way of telling me that my eagerness to learn our findings was disruptive. She said, "What you're asking me to do is akin to pulling up a vegetable every day to see if it's growing." This is the tendency of most Americans, so inundated with fast-breaking news that we despise waiting, so disturbed by even the most remote threat that we never fully relax, so accustomed to an incessant torrent of mental enticements that our attention spans are constantly shrinking.

This is a cycle we must break. When we marinate our minds in negativity and fear, we spur both the nocebo effect and the fight-or-flight response, which have detrimental effects on our bodies and cause us more worry. Over a lifetime of viewing commercials in which pain relievers save the day, we come to overrely on pain relievers, only to become convinced we have other ailments that require other drugs. The more extreme or outlandish the information we come to absorb and accept, the higher ratings and sales are reported, the more the media will try to feed our frenzy. And as John Updike suggested, we'll never make "enough" part of our vocabulary.

Is it possible to break this cycle? We cannot rely on those in charge of dispensing information to modify their messages. Since Hollywood hasn't turned away from violent or explicit programming, parents have resorted to installing V-chips in their televisions to prevent children from viewing inappropriate shows. But our brains don't need V-chips. Wonderfully, humans already have a custom-installed device that filters information we receive and that can be empowered to heal us. This device is your belief system—the thoughts, feelings, and values that are unique to you and your life experiences. Our minds are conditioned to react in certain ways, the wiring of our brains formed when we repeatedly call upon particular memories or thoughts and their signature neurons and neuron combinations.

Because the brain is ever-changing, we have the ability to rewire and modify those automatic reactions in a process sometimes called "cognitive restructuring." In fact, *the very act of reading these words*—the brain processing, incorporating, and integrating their meaning—is forever changing your brain's wiring. Every new experience, every new fact entered into your brain changes its configuration and your awareness and understanding of who you were, who you are, and who you will be. Because of the brain's intrinsic malleability, you have the opportunity to literally "change your mind."

In all the activities I am about to recommend, the goal is not to deny reality, only to project images and ideas of something better for yourself. You act "as if" the preferred reality were true and the body responds. Writer Sherry Suib Cohen shares her version of "acting as if" in a book called *Secrets of a Very Good Marriage: Lessons from the Sea*. In it she describes how desperately her husband wanted her to love their boat, to lavish it with "unqualified reverence" despite the fact that if it were not for her husband's passion for fishing, this boat was one of the last places she'd ever hope to be. She writes, "But, if truth be told, I felt foolish praising an imperfect boat with such glowing strokes. In my heart it was an okay, far-from-perfect boat: Why shouldn't I tell the entire and absolute truth?" Suib Cohen goes on to suggest that marriages are nourished by audible strokes because "speaking love out loud and often enough makes love invincible."

The same is true of our bodies. As much time as we devote in our lives to "the entire and absolute truth"—which may not be the true picture but rather an unduly negative interpretation—our brains and bodies need to indulge occasionally in brighter possibilities. By acting as if our bodies are invincible in the ways I'll prescribe, greater health can emerge.

Automatic Thoughts

You'll want to start by identifying negative automatic reactions—the unrealistic, irrational, or distorted thoughts that cause stress. *The Wellness Book,* which I wrote together with my long-standing colleague Eileen M. Stewart, RN, C, MS, and other members of the Mind/Body Medical Institute, offers a much more comprehensive approach to breaking these habits. In it, Dr. Ann Webster, together with Ms. Stewart and Ms. Carol L. Wells-Federman, state:

> Cognitive restructuring does not gloss over or deny negative feelings or distress—there are many things in our lives over which it is appropriate to feel anxious, depressed, angry, frustrated, etc. . . . What we emphasize is paying attention to how our thoughts influence our feelings in order to avoid *excessive* or automatic anxiety, depression, anger, guilt, etc., so that these emotions are not the only way you feel. When governed by strong emotions, *the mind becomes a filter, letting into consciousness only those thoughts that reinforce that mood.* Little else is allowed through.

We are all constantly talking to ourselves, engaging an internal chatterbox in which we critique, advise, bolster, and dream about ourselves. After saying something enough times, we start to believe it. If you tell yourself, "I'm unattractive," or "My body fails me," enough times, these thoughts become "realities" for you.

Eleanor Roosevelt once said, "No one can make you feel inferior without your consent." This is profoundly true because a steady stream of self-doubting thoughts erodes one's confidence, the very confidence you need to project to the world and that your body needs to remember wellness. To compound the problem, we develop what Dr. Donald Meichenbaum of the University of Waterloo calls a "confirmatory bias" in which we seek out only the information, people, and situations that match our mood and feelings of self-worth. To break this chain of events, you must change your internal dialogue.

In *The Wellness Book*, we recommend this exercise. The next time you are stuck in traffic and you feel your blood pressure rising, try this:

- Stop
- Breathe and release physical tension
- Reflect and ask yourself these questions:
  What's going on here?
  Why am I so distressed?
  Am I late, or am I just racing against time?
  Is it really a crisis that I'm late?
  If I am late, what is the worst thing that will happen?
  Will worrying about it help?
- Choose not to think so anxiously

Talking back to ourselves in this way, with this four-step process—Stop; Breathe and release physical tension; Reflect; and Choose—we can diminish and eventually break ourselves of automatic reactions. We can limit the negativity that stressful situations inspire, changing the opinions and moods that conspire in our brains/bodies to affect our health.

Visualizations and Affirmations

Another important strategy for rewiring the brain and redirecting your internal dialogue is to counter the usual onslaught of negativity with visualizations and affirmations, the same techniques I mentioned earlier in the book.

Buddhists make very active use of visualizations to rid themselves of anger and bitterness. In one meditation, they envision images of themselves being superimposed on their worst
enemies. Because it is too difficult to maintain anger when we
recognize parts of ourselves in the actions and visage of others, this kind of visualization works very well.

We too can take advantage of the top-down thinking that
makes visualizations very powerful in our minds/bodies.
You'll recall how, in illustrations that appeared (in Figures 5
and 6) earlier in the book, when a woman saw a beautiful pastoral scene and recalled it later, she triggered the same wiring
in her brain. It's very easy to incorporate this wisdom into a
meditative technique, using as a focus a mountain stream,
great work of art, or any other favorite, soothing scene.

As I covered in my book *Your Maximum Mind*, athletes frequently use visualizations in their training. They learn to elicit
the relaxation response and then visualize, over and over,
their ideal performance. With this, they wire themselves, so at
the time of the competition their minds and bodies can play
out these wired configurations.

You'll recall that affirmations are, simply, positive
thoughts—short phrases or sayings that mean something to
you. They work the same way that commercials dreamed up
by top-dollar Madison Avenue advertising agencies work. The
top-down repetition of these healthy messages becomes a part
of your internal dialogue, a theme that changes your belief
system and rewires your brain. Our patients find them particularly effective when used right after eliciting the relaxation
response, when the mind is quiet and receptive. Here are
some examples:

- "I can handle it."
- "I accept myself as I am."
- "I am peaceful."
- "I am becoming healthy and strong."
- "Let it be."
- "I am doing the best that I can."

Humor

Of course, as well as affirmations work, they're also the brunt of many jokes on *Saturday Night Live*, which brings us to one of the most effective medicines of all in combating negativity—humor. Dr. George E. Vaillant of Harvard Medical School wrote in his book *Adaptation to Life:*

> Humor is one of the truly elegant defenses in the human repertoire. Few would deny that the capacity for humor, like hope, is one of mankind's most potent antidotes for the woes of Pandora's box.

Humor, smiles, and laughter are the very best stress-busters. In *The Wellness Book*, colleagues Margaret BaiM, MS, RN, and comedian Loretta LaRoche, BA, all but recommend that everyone concerned for their health purchase not pills, self-help manuals, or exercise mats, but Groucho Marx glasses. Donning a big nose, bushy mustache, and spiderlike eyebrows, little seems wrong with the world. Or when you count your blessings, when you force yourself to recount joys rather than sorrows, fun rather than gloom, silliness rather than stodginess, your thoughts will settle into delight and your body will respond.

Healthy Distractions

I also urge you to lead a life of healthy distraction. Engage your mind and your energies in helping others and in caring for a world that desperately needs an injection of hope. A May 1995 Associated Press article reports that 47 percent of American children say they have dismal expectations for their futures. About 53 percent fear poverty, 50 percent fear kidnapping, 45 percent physical or sexual abuse. A ten-year-old respondent, Janelle, told researchers, "I'm scared of being killed. I want to live my life to the fullest and do everything. I don't want to be dead."

One should not try to candy-coat Janelle's world. If she's surrounded by violence, poverty, and chaos in her neighborhood, she'll have to struggle to survive, not just to maintain her hopes and aspirations. Drug abuse and senseless violence are enormous threats to public health, and we must not gloss over the gravity of the situation, but try to alleviate it so that hope and its healing effects can be restored.

Obviously, there's a whole world in need of our attention. We've already seen with Alan Luks's evidence of the helper's high that one of the healthiest things you can do for yourself is to volunteer to help your community, backing away from too much self-worry and fretting. Focusing our attention away from our own problems by helping others, we can experience physical benefits, instead of passively absorbing a deluge of bad news, panic, and fear—the physical translation of which is very damaging.

Learning to Let Go

In balancing the stresses and information overload of life, I believe it's valuable to adopt this approach: Gather all the pertinent information, make a decision, and then "let go" of it. Allow time for the new facts to be incorporated in your brain, and to change your wiring and the way you perceive yourself and life. Our brain physiology makes the adage "Sleep on it" very pragmatic. In fact, dreaming is believed to represent the time in which the brain is rearranging and rewiring itself. Consolidation of thoughts and memories occurs, and the bizarre twists and images of our dreams often represent the processing and reclassifying of old information.

Eliciting the relaxation response may work much the same way. Often after people finish meditating, they view the world differently, through "new eyes." Many people report increased creativity after eliciting the relaxation response, which makes sense given that creativity is often simply an act of interpreting the same facts in different ways.

All the strategies I've proposed can help you register new and powerful beliefs in your brain, brightening your mood, and making information and news you receive less apt to hurt or bother you. Nevertheless, when illness is involved, it's very hard to let go, laugh off, affirm away, or talk back to a diagnosis.

My collaborator on this book, Marg Stark, had to learn to let go of a focus on illness. The summer after she graduated from Mount Holyoke College, Marg was rushed into surgery for an abundance of large, abdominal growths a gynecologist found during a routine checkup. When she awakened after the operation, an intern abruptly informed her that her condition did not appear to be cancerous but that she had a severe case of endometriosis. Her doctor later told her that it was the worst case he had seen in a woman so young, speculating that she had less than a 30 percent chance of being able to conceive children.

With the prospect of infertility thrust upon her at age twenty-two when her writing career, not marriage and children, was foremost on her mind, Marg began to educate herself about endometriosis and its treatment. Although much mystery remains about the cause of the condition, endometriosis occurs when the endometrium, or the lining of the uterus, appears outside the uterus, causing monthly internal bleeding and subsequent inflammation of tissues, which can clump together and apply pressure to or block other organs. Endometriosis is chronic, ceasing only with pregnancy and menopause.

When Marg was diagnosed, endometriosis was still often referred to as "the career woman's disease." It was so dubbed because physicians who first became familiar with the condition developed a profile of typical endometriosis patients—namely, highly ambitious, Caucasian women who put off having children to pursue careers. A significant misinterpretation, the profile was later abandoned when physicians began seeing the disease in women of considerable diversity. For years, many women with endometriosis went undiagnosed because doctors dismissed or belittled the menstrual pain these women reported, which is often the only early symptom of the condition. Presumably, white career women who had more access to the medical system were just more determined in pursuing diagnosis and treatment.

Like the women who blame themselves for breast cancer, Marg began blaming herself for a lifestyle that she thought had brought on a condition that might make her barren. She began to question the training she'd received at a high-powered women's college, which encouraged her to combine career and family, and she worried about the wisdom of taking on the stressful demands of a newspaper reporter's career. The daughter of a Presbyterian minister, Marg also began to question her faith, that despite her deep desire for children, this might not be "God's will." On top of these emotional adjustments, she endured weight gain, hot flashes, night sweats, and other miserable side effects of a synthetic male hormone she took to stem the disease.

But with time, Marg let go of what she admits became an inappropriate fixation on endometriosis and potential infertility. She decided that if her legacy to the world was not to be children, she wanted it to be her writing. She left behind the endometriosis support group that had been very helpful to her in the beginning but that later began to revive her fears and led her to focus on the disease. She decided that God was good, and that while no theology seemed to adequately address her questions, maybe there were some mysteries in life that she was not supposed to solve. She sought out highly recommended endometriosis specialists and up-and-coming treatments but, except for a greater appreciation for the need to manage stress in her life, Marg left her anxieties about endometriosis to her doctors.

Ten years have gone by and Marg has no more apparent growth of endometriosis. Married last year, she and her husband plan to have children, either biologically or by adoption. Still, had she known then what she knows today about mind/body connections, self-care, and the importance of her outlook, Marg believes it would not have taken so long to let go of the burden of her diagnosis. As I've said before, the power of diagnosis is immense. But I've come to understand that our minds and our belief systems, the filter through which diagnoses and all information in life are screened, can, as John Milton wrote in *Paradise Lost*, "make a Heaven of Hell, a Hell of Heaven."

The suggestions I've offered here may help you change your mind, and your reality. And in the next chapter, I'll share the life lessons I've garnered in my search for something that lasts. By incorporating these wisdoms, medicine, society, and individuals themselves may at last be able to fully appreciate and enjoy the rich interplay of our minds, bodies, and souls. In this interplay is a timeless, unending source of healing.

CHAPTER 13

TIMELESS HEALING

There is a source of healing that lasts. Progress in medical research will never dull or overthrow the intrinsic truth of remembered wellness. Heraclitus, the fifth-century B.C. Greek philosopher, is credited with saying, "Nothing endures but change." But after thirty years of research, I'm ready to counter that claim and to say that faith itself is enduring, transcending all the changes wrought by time and fate. This is the solace I offer to you in light of the fact that this book has suggested hefty amounts of change for Western society, medicine, and for individuals themselves. I recognize that the terms I've used and the changes I'm recommending can be daunting: "remembering wellness," "rewiring the brain," "believing in an Infinite Absolute," "trusting instincts," "exercising beliefs," and "letting go."

It is precisely because change, for the better or for the worse, is stress-inducing that I will devote this last chapter to commonsense steps you can take to change your perspective and to live more healthfully. Making practical use of remembered wellness, the faith factor, and other forms of self-care, we, as individuals, can restructure our thinking for better health, maybe even for a better world.

An Overhaul of Western Thinking

Change is inevitable. These findings could result in an overhaul of Western medicine and science. The guiding principles of the existing health care system will have to be changed, but we will be fiddling with what is already very good medicine. The medical profession is already under considerable strain, trying to cope with the many problems of health care financing, personnel and resource cutbacks, unprecedented competition, consolidation of services, and regulatory change. Moreover, the profession is challenged to care for people whose problems—poverty, violence, or the ravages of HIV—we cannot yet cure.

Mind/body medical advocates are also asking busy and often stressed individuals to add yet another layer of responsibility to their lives and schedules. Undoubtedly, individuals will have to assume a greater share of their medical decision-making, spend more time pursuing remembered wellness, get up earlier in the morning, or find one more window of time in their schedules for eliciting the relaxation response. But perhaps most profoundly we are asking people to protect themselves against another newly identified public health threat, to position themselves against the tide of Western thought, and to think in ways that seem contrary to what they've been taught.

But here's the saving grace. The term "remember" is the key to soothing anxieties about all this change. Your body, like all the human bodies on the planet and all that have come before you, is designed to remember and revive health and well-being. It is not as if you have to start from scratch. You don't have to build a new brain, a new body, or a new soul; they are intrinsically designed to rebuild themselves.

You have always had a resource within you to affect your health, whether or not you made optimal use of it. And your brain is malleable enough that it's possible to restructure your thinking and the neurosignatures that, over time, recruit nerve cells in your brain to conduct your usual thoughts and actions. As long as you understand that the effects are cumulative, there is no thought or knee-jerk emotional reaction too ingrained for you to alter. It may take time, as it did for the brain to feel the impact of repeated negativity or pessimism. But as we've seen, the time is time well spent. Remembered wellness can be very transforming, even lifesaving.

Furthermore, beliefs and faith have enjoyed a very healthy counterculture existence. Of course, objective fact has been worshiped in public realms. But privately, the human spirit with its inexorable links to human physiology has never allowed faith, hope, and love—the cravings of the soul—to be obliterated. No society has ever banished them, no people ever lived without them. They are eternal, natural inclinations that modern Western thought has suppressed but never subdued.

The Implications and Opportunities

As a physician, I am not qualified to address all the implications mind/body medicine may have on society and its mores. And I leave it to spiritual and religious leaders to decide how religious communities and mainline traditions will assimilate this information. But my patients have taught me a great deal about the opportunities that emerge when artificial barriers are broken down, about how physical ailments inspire soul-searching and a revival of meaningful living, and about how the human spirit enlivens and transforms the body. And my sense is that physicians and pastors, scientists and religious believers, health enthusiasts and the spiritually inclined have far more in common than we typically think, insights that, when shared and exchanged, could help transform humankind. Indeed, remembered wellness offers more opportunities than threats.

So how far might remembered wellness and other mind/body approaches go in transforming the world as we know it? The potential of the human spirit is staggering. Instinctively, we've always known this. Our wiring ensured that we knew it. Our brain's reliance on emotion to sort and prioritize inputs has always ensured that emotionally and spiritually laden beliefs had considerable say in the determination of our health. But as much as we've sensed the power of the human will, having scientific confirmation of the power is all the more impressive, at least to the Western way of thinking. Now we have scientific permission to champion what we've always privately believed.

But what are the best ways for society to champion the cause of the visceral human soul? How is it healthy for society to implement remembered wellness? My colleagues and I have conducted several studies in which the elicitation of the relaxation response was incorporated into high school curricula. We found that high school sophomores who were taught to elicit the response had significantly higher levels of self-esteem than did their peers who were not exposed to training about the relaxation response. Furthermore, our studies showed that students liked using the relaxation response, and there were reports from teachers of decreased inappropriate classroom behaviors among students who had learned the mental focusing techniques. Under the leadership of Ms. Wilcher, teams from the Mind/Body Medical Institute are presently at work further evaluating the effects of the relaxation response, this time in schools in Massachusetts, New Jersey, and California.

We've also introduced many corporations and workplaces to the relaxation response and our other stress-management techniques with very positive results. The John Hancock Insurance Company, Perini Corporation, and the Houghton Mifflin publishing company are just a few of the corporations that have asked the Mind/Body Medical Institute to teach their workers mental focusing techniques. With job stress being a major contributor to illness, and with illness costing businesses billions of dollars in insurance reimbursement, workman's compensation, sick days, and general loss of productivity, colleagues Ms. Wilcher and Richard Dalton have found the private sector, government, the armed services, and many other employers are eager to learn the low-cost, big-dividend wisdoms of the relaxation response and remembered wellness.

In a 1993 article in *Business Week*, George Bennett, the president of the Lexington, Massachusetts, consulting firm Symetrix, said the reason he hired the Mind/Body Medical Institute to teach his employees the merits of self-care was that employees so often complained of being stressed out. "There's no question employees who do this are more relaxed, and some are even more productive," he says. One of his employees, a diabetic, experienced a 15 percent decrease in the insulin he needed after using the relaxation techniques for three weeks.

An article from *Fortune* magazine entitled "Leaders Learn to Heed the Voice Within" described how, increasingly, major companies are touting the art of "reflection" in the "fast-moving New Economy." Business schools from Harvard to the

University of California are also getting into the act, teaching burgeoning business leaders to "heed the voice within."

Inner Peace, Outer Peace

There's no question in my mind that no matter where self-care habits are taught in American society, they will foster a healthier, calmer, and more productive populace. But I worry about using these principles of science to bolster specific types of meditation or specific theologies. I believe that when it comes to garnering the full measure of remembered wellness with mental focusing techniques, the teacher should not impose views on the student. We need to be aware that "appropriateness to the individual" empowers these mechanisms within the body. Certainly, science can find "commonalties" among people, for example, that we all respond to human touch, or that we often find rituals meaningful. But we cannot, for example, make aromatherapy work for someone who isn't inclined, or wired, to respond to it. There isn't one affirmation that will restructure everyone's thinking for the better, nor will "Lord Jesus Christ, have mercy on me" be a very satisfying means of eliciting the relaxation response for, say, someone who's Jewish.

As researchers learn more about emotion and its crucial contribution to brain function, we must keep in mind that we all still operate with different emotions and strengths of emotions. As we saw in the ethnocentric studies of pain, our diversity makes us perceive pain differently, emotionally and thus physically. We will never be wired to entertain the same beliefs, or one particular faith.

The Relaxation Response in the Schools?

Many people could read the facts that I've presented here—the evidence that mind, body, and soul are mingled—and believe that a separation of church and state is therefore impossible and inappropriate. Again, I am a physician and not a public policy-maker. My position is to point out the win-win situations that are possible in health. For example, it is conceivable that children in public schools could be taught to elicit the physiologic benefits of the relaxation response and that the students who wanted to could apply their religious beliefs to evoke remembered wellness as well, the health benefits of which are proven and which I have identified as the faith factor. Schools could set aside a period of silence during which children could practice this habit, some of them using a secular focus to elicit the relaxation response purely for its health benefits, some eliciting it with prayer, and still others declining to do it at all. Thus, the health and self-esteem benefits could be promoted, and people could exercise their beliefs in ways that are meaningful to them.

But at the same time, it would run counter to the evidence I've gathered for diverse children and diverse people in a public setting to be taught that any one technique, or any one set of beliefs, would reap universal physical rewards. To enjoy the health benefits of remembered wellness, you have to heed your own instincts, appreciating the unique set of life experiences and emotions contained in the neurosignatures of your brain. The meaning you afford to your life, the healing trust you place in a caregiver, or the solace you grasp from a belief in an Infinite Absolute is uniquely powerful for you.

As subjective as remembered wellness is, there are some definitive things I can say about incorporating healing beliefs and faith into your life. These are some of the principles and practical lessons I've drawn from my long medical quest for lasting truths. I hope they prove helpful to you:

1. Practice and apply self-care regularly.

Work with your doctor, and with unconventional practitioners if you so choose, to learn self-care habits, the neglected leg of the three-legged stool. I consider self-care anything an individual can do, independent of doctors or healers, to enhance his or her health. This includes mind/body reactions such as remembered wellness, the relaxation response, and the faith factor. It also embraces good nutrition, exercise, and other means of stress management.

You'll recall that in Chapter 12 I highlighted self-care tactics such as affirmations, visualizations, a hearty sense of humor, healthy distractions, and letting go of anxiety. And earlier in the book, I talked about the health benefits of religious activity, music, rituals, friendship and socializing, human touch, prayer, and volunteer work. When you make these kinds of activities and commitments a locus of your life, you'll *feel* and you'll be healthier. I don't mean to make light of a difficult reality you face, but if you conceive more for yourself than you would normally, your mind/body will, to a certain extent, respond as if the ideal were possible. With this approach, seemingly unachievable events can be achieved.

I use the term "self-care" because it puts the onus on you, it shifts the emphasis from your role as passive patient to active participant, a shift that medicine has not always encouraged. However, as you will recall, I caution against becoming self-absorbed in self-care. Don't become fixated on your health or on the avoidance of aging, illness, or death. Make your daily elicitation of the relaxation response, your jog, or your salad at lunch a no-brainer, which you do not analyze or overthink. Simply delight in the event itself in all the ways that you can.

If you don't have enough of these soul-nourishing pleasures in your life, or if you don't know where to begin, you'll find a magnitude of resources available to you in any library, bookstore, church/synagogue newsletter, adult education promotional, community bulletin board, or computer on-line bulletin board. Just remember to modify information according to your belief system, your gut instincts, and the experiences unique to you. If they're marketed well, exercise videos, self-help books, spirituality lectures, religious retreats, get-rich schemes, and mind/body messages will play on your emotions, making you believe that you can't live without them, or that your life will be changed overnight with their influence.

Remember that change in our lives, because of our wiring and conditioned responses, is gradual and cumulative. So extract the gems or slivers of truth that your belief system advocates, then let the other advice slide off your back. You are, after all, the authority on living your life.

Since the vast majority of the medical complaints brought to doctors' offices are stress- and belief-related, you must learn to care for and heal yourself most of the time. Don't be alarmed by this prospect. Your body already does this day in, day out, and is astoundingly good at it.

Again, it's almost always valuable to seek the assistance of your physician to determine the difference between a condition that will benefit from self-care exclusively and one that requires the other two legs of the stool—drugs or procedures—to treat. Learning about your body and its ebb and flow is an evolutionary process. You'll work toward a more independent attitude. Become acquainted with the warning signs of heart attacks, strokes, cancer, and other life-threatening diseases. Over time, you'll develop a sense of what symptoms are important—those that are extreme or don't go away.

As I've said, I'm not suggesting that you become maniacally alert or preoccupied with every ache or pain. Sensible monitoring of bodily change is the key. When a woman is taught to examine her breasts in monthly self-exams, she learns that the most important thing to look for is change. Practicing self-exams, a woman comes to know her particular contours, tissue, and cycle so that she will recognize new sensations, indentations, or growths. This is a sage example for us in observing our overall health. If you're accustomed and attuned to your body's normal, everyday function in which minor aches and pains are common, in which a stressful day is apt to bring on a headache or a certain food triggers digestion problems, you'll be better able to spot an unusual reaction. Respecting this maintenance routine inside of you, perhaps you'll be obliged to feed it more healthfully, to rest when you need to, to exercise this wonderful machine and support it with a positive life outlook.

How influential can a coordinated contingent of self-care

habits be? We honestly don't know, but Dr. Dean Ornish, president of the Preventive Medicine Research Institute in Sausalito, California, found that heart disease could not only be relieved but *reversed* when patients made significant changes in diet, exercise, and stress management. Our two programs will soon be compared in a groundbreaking research project sponsored by the Commonwealth of Massachusetts Group Insurance Commission and the John Hancock Insurance Company. In this comparison, patients with heart disease will be divided between our two clinics in hopes that we can gauge the adherence to and results of various self-care components and other treatments. Explorations such as this will help medicine prescribe revolutionary change for itself, heightening the respect physicians have for patient-empowered healing.

It would also be interesting to study Christian Scientists who eschew all medical care except dentistry and bone setting. Does faith alone make them well? Is there something to learn from a community that relies on faith, not pills and procedures?

2. Know your truth.

Each of us possesses an awesome healing power. It takes your belief to imbue the caregiver and the treatment with the power of remembered wellness. So whenever you get medical advice, no matter what the source, hold fast to the scientifically proven power that you wield.

You'll recall the story in which Antonia Baquero, who had a previous scare with a precancerous condition, panicked after a Chinese healer with impaired judgment told her she didn't look well. In these situations, it's critical to remember that you are an authority on what will hurt or heal you. Don't let any physician or healer, fortune-teller or card reader, preacher or teacher, magazine story or medical book, friend or lover, therapist or support group impress something untrue upon you.

Truth, like scientific fact, is supposed to be unassailable. But the truth buried in minds, bodies, and souls is often a cache of meaning and joy far more substantial than the truth of a diagnosis, label, category, or statistic. Some of the most inspiring people I've ever met are those who, despite AIDS or diseases for which no cure is known, carry on with purposefulness and humor, verve and compassion, not allowing their disease to overcome their souls. The Bible says that the truth will set us free, and often when we find it deep within ourselves, it can.

3. Beware of people with all the answers.

Be careful of any physician, nontraditional healer, spiritual guide, mind/body guru, or any adviser who claims to have all the answers, or wants others to think so. Besides love and sex, writers and lecturers today take up few topics with as much evangelistic zeal as health and spirituality. It will be no small task shielding these very personal matters from unhealthy speculation and overanalysis, but start with tuning out overly confident or all-knowing mentors and guides. Value your emotions and intuitions the same way your brain does; don't let someone manipulate your wiring for their gain.

Karen Armstrong suggested in *A History of God* that mysticism pursued in prayer might be dangerous without the aid of a trustworthy guide. So too have charismatic leaders throughout history, politicians and dictators, cult figures and champions of justice, appealed to people by telling them what they wanted to hear. Mind/body medicine should remind us of the precious nature of our minds, and of the importance of critiquing the messages we allow to become actualized in our brains/bodies.

Having visited the grand and seemingly perfect Taj Mahal on my travels to India, I was told that the architect explicitly designed the building to have one minor flaw—a tiny leak in the roof! In that day, rulers so despised the notion that their palaces might in any way be copied or duplicated that architects worried they would be murdered upon completion of royal projects. Consequently, some suggest, this architect left something within the structure undone and unperfected so that his services would continue to be in demand. Still others say the architect wanted the flaw built into the structure to remind humans to honor the fact that only God is capable of perfection.

Whether or not you believe in God, I believe that we are all wired to crave meaning in life, to assign profound power and sacredness to human experiences, and sometimes even to lend "god" status or "godliness" to humans and human endeavors. Be wary of this tendency, because it may rob spiritual life of its mysterious grandeur, of the wonderful transcendent qualities that cannot be accessed entirely by human intellect, and because it makes us very susceptible to human manipulation. Not only is your body a temple, but your mind is an architect, busy transforming the ideas and inspirations you feed it. Protect it from those who exploit the power of remembered wellness for their own gain.

4. Remember the nocebo is equally powerful.

Unfortunately, remembered wellness has a flip side. Monkey mind may inappropriately trigger the fight-or-flight response in the body. Similarly, automatic negative thoughts, bad moods, and compulsive worrying eventually take up physical residence in our bodies. Extreme examples of the nocebo effect include voodoo death, belief-engendered death, mass psychogenic illness, false memories, and "memories" of alien abductions. People who dwell on worst-case scenarios, who exaggerate risks, or who project doubt and undue worry keep the nocebo effect busy in their physiology. They signal their brains to send help when no physical sickness is present, persuading the body to get sick when there is no biologic reason sickness should occur.

Furthermore, the nocebo effect thrives in American culture. The illusion of ideal beauty and perfect health taunts us, often committing us to a treadmill of dissatisfaction and insecurity. Advertisers promote this mentality so we need their clients' products when, in fact, our bodies are already amazingly equipped and steeled against illness and injury. Medicine too has lost its awe for the body's healing prowess and has become unreasonably intolerant of all symptoms and overly impressed with its own therapeutic tools.

With remembered wellness, I am not suggesting that everyone needs to become Alfred E. Neuman or Little Mary Sunshine. Fate is sometimes very unkind, our burdens and challenges enormous. But tremendous wisdom and inordinate physical healing lie in a prayer composed by the American theologian Reinhold Niebuhr: "O God, give us the serenity to accept what cannot be changed, courage to change things that should be changed, and wisdom to distinguish the one from the other."

I'm sometimes asked if it's healthy for curmudgeons and pessimists, who know no other way to cope than to thrive on anxiety and negative thinking, to change to a more affirmative lifestyle. Again, you have to find beliefs that work for you, and what's great progress in one person may feel like baby steps to another. However slight, it's always dramatic and wonderful to witness the springing forth of happiness and peace in a formerly obstinate spirit. Even in these extreme cases, I believe a modicum of change is beneficial, both emotionally and physically.

5. Trust your instincts more often.

In "Pragmatism," a lecture he delivered in 1907, William James wrote, "The philosophy which is important in each of us is not a technical matter; it is our more or less dumb sense of what life honestly and deeply means. It is only partly got from books; it is our individual way of just seeing and feeling the total push and pressure of the cosmos."

People describe the process of finding out what is important to them, of tapping into their beliefs, in very different ways, sometimes calling it "soul-searching," "mulling it over," "listening to one's heart," "going inside of one's self," "praying," or "sleeping on it." Some people act on instincts or common sense; others find a truth or intuition emerges slowly. But most people know when something "feels right." Most people have a kind of internal radar that occasionally calls out to them.

The next time you're faced with a major decision, medical or otherwise, ask yourself, "What feels like the right thing to do?," or "What would I do if the choice were entirely up to me?" I'm not suggesting that you make decisions based on this factor alone, but at least let belief be a player. Honor your convictions and perceptions enough to make them a part of a hearty intellectual argument.

Our conditioning, from Descartes on, has been to cordon off emotion from reason, fact from opinion, even though we now are learning that objectivity is subjective, and that reason relies on emotion. To gear our beliefs and emotions to work for us, we have to listen to them more than typical Western and American upbringings have trained us to do.

In his book on synesthesia, you'll recall that Dr. Cytowic remarks that we all know more than we think we know. And because, as he says, "emotion has a logic of its own" and is so instrumental in assigning priorities of thoughts and impressions in our brains, we would be wise to start paying more attention to our emotions and beliefs. But in deciding between the Western world's view and our own internal view, he writes:

> The first step in breaking through to the transcendent is putting aside the idea that we have to choose between objective and subjective views of reality. Many aspects of human experience cannot be conveyed by objective facts, nor is there any escape from subjectivity. In addition to a detached, objective view based on externals and a subjective view based on our inner life, there is a third choice grounded in experience, through which noetic understanding is found. This is the depth at which we really live.

Taking that third choice, you can mingle objective observations with emotions and gut reactions. If after hearing everything a surgeon has to say, the prospect of facial surgery and having half of your jaw removed to eliminate a tumor is more abhorrent to you than death, as it was for Barbara Dawson, you need not apologize for this conviction. If you've carefully weighed your options and decided you'd rather skip red meat and other animal products the rest of your life than have open-heart surgery, this is your right. And you'd be wise to practice your right, after gathering all the information, surrounding yourself with physicians and caregivers you trust, and filtering the facts through the belief system you've acquired over a lifetime of your unique experiences.

We'd all prefer there to be right and wrong answers, hard and fast information, and no-load, risk-free health care solutions. But no such clear-cut world exists. Health need not be pursued by hunches, but the most that any good doctor, together with an informed patient, can do is offer an educated guess or a best estimate. In developing this best estimate, we'd all be wise to listen to the body more often and to regard our beliefs with greater respect.

Let your instincts guide you. Follow them up with research. Put your health in good, trustworthy hands. Let your health have time to correct itself. Invest remembered wellness and a reasonable application of self-care, medications, and surgery for maximum health returns.

6. Remember that immortality is impossible.

While it's healthy to listen to your heart, it's also harmful to deny or duck the truth. No one lives forever. No matter how well-versed you become in mind/body medicine, no matter how far medical progress may be able to set back the clock, death is, like illness and pain, an unfortunate but natural fact of life.

I must sound as if I'm talking in circles, first telling you not to let a diagnosis define you, then warning you not to fall prey to denial. Nonetheless, some lecturers and New Age entrepreneurs imply that all disease is curable and that we can avoid death and aging if we only believe. These salesmen do great harm to people by fostering guilt, and damage the field of mind/body medicine, which is legitimately trying to establish its findings and change the way Western medicine is practiced. No evidence exists that death can be denied its eventual toll.

There's a wonderful scene in the movie *Moonstruck* in which actress Olympia Dukakis, playing a wife who knows her husband is cheating on her, leans across a table in an intimate Italian restaurant to ask her male companion a long-festering question, "Why do men chase women?" Giving Olympia Dukakis's character the answer she knows in her heart is true, he replies, "Because we fear death?" Indeed, fear of death can bring out the worst in people, but the realization that death is an inevitable, natural occurrence can also propel healthy, impassioned living.

It's a subtle distinction. We often use the phrase "living as if there were no tomorrow," "as if" becoming an important, albeit subtle, truth. Living well, exercising and eating appropriately, seeing doctors when you need to but not overrelying on the medical system, these are all proven buffers against disease and illness.

7. Let faith, the ultimate belief, heal you.

St. Anselm, who is believed to have lived between 1033 and 1109, wrote, "God is that, the greater than which cannot be conceived." Belief in God, in the ultimate conceivable greatness, is the most influential form of remembered wellness. With death a loathsome destiny, we cherish a better explanation of life. Whether we "remember" the peace of God because God wants us to, or we "remember" a life-transcending power because our evolution made it a requisite for survival, faith in a supreme being is a supreme physical healer.

According to medical research, faith in God is good for us, and this benefit is not exclusive to one denomination or theology. You can believe in God in a quiet, introspective way, or declare your convictions out loud to the world, and still reap the physiologic rewards.

For many reasons, religious activity and churchgoing is also healthy. Religious groups encourage all kinds of health-affirming activities, fellowship and socializing perhaps first among them, but also prayer, volunteerism, familiar rituals, and music. Prayer, in particular, appears to be therapeutic, the specifics of which science will continue to explore.

I find that sometimes people are reluctant to rely on faith to soothe them. They think religion is a crutch and they don't like to think they need it. And I've heard others disparage the "last-minute conversions" that often occur in people who are seriously ill. But the truth of the matter is that faith is a natural and inevitable physiologic reaction to the threats to mortality we all face. We cannot help but be drawn to it in an hour of need. In II Corinthians 12:9, the apostle Paul describes the Lord's reply to his appeals for relief from a physical ailment, saying, "My grace is all you need, for my power is strongest when you are weak."

I believe that humans are wired for faith and that there is a special healing generated by people who rely on faith. So whether or not you believe in God per se, try to conceive of greatness beyond which there can be nothing greater.

8. Respect others' beliefs. Don't impose yours.

You may recall the Old Testament story of the Tower of Babel. Explaining how the tower got its name, Genesis 11:9 tells us, "Therefore its name was called Babel, because there the Lord confused the language of all the earth; and from there the Lord scattered them abroad over the face of all the earth." Before that time, the Bible says, all humans spoke the same language and, trying to aggrandize and make names for themselves, built a city on a mountaintop and a tower that reached into the heavens. At Pentecost, Christians celebrate the reversal of Babel's linguistic disaster—a fiery-fingered spirit that came upon the apostles after Christ's resurrection and enabled believers of many different languages and cultures to speak in the same tongue.

It is human nature to "name" and distinguish things in the world around us. But often we seem far more interested in the things that divide and distinguish us from one another than the things we share in common. Similarly in science, we reduce the grand human experience to smaller and smaller physical components, without appreciating enduring truths or wonderful commonalties among people.

Studies of remembered wellness have persuaded me that, coincidentally or by divine decree, humans do have a universal, physical propensity for faith. At our core, we are all organisms sustained and nourished by life-affirming beliefs and philosophies. We are designed to flex spiritual muscles, even if our prayers are very different, even if we don't call it prayer. Scattered across the globe, in nearly every culture and time known to us, people have said prayers and meditations that evoked physiological calm, or the relaxation response. No matter how confused our languages, no matter how distinct our cultures and creeds, we share innate gifts—of physical healing, of achieving peace, and sometimes of feeling "the presence of a power of energy force which feels near."

I believe there's something substantially true about Karen Armstrong's exhortation that it's dangerous for people to "personalize" God. My research has shown that the mysterious, transcendent, and intuitive experience of God is very powerful, and that Western society and medicine often do a great deal of harm to the human spirit by focusing on specifics rather than the big picture. We end up taking away from the awe-inspiring truth, that the mind and the body are remarkably good at keeping us well, and that all of us share these healing properties in common.

Barbara Dawson, the woman who I told you chose radiation and prayer over an operation to remove the cancer from her face and neck, tells me that immediately after I left her room at Beth Israel Hospital in Boston where she was hospitalized— where I taught her to elicit the relaxation response for the first time—she wanted to share her experience with others.

"I was on a spiritual high, not an overwhelming feeling, just a very peaceful, loving feeling, and I said to myself, 'I have to share this with somebody,'" she explains. "I walked down the hall and I saw a lady sitting by the window in her room, so I walked in slowly and I introduced myself. She was very welcoming to me, we exchanged recipes and stories about our grandchildren. And she was telling me that she had cancer and that she was petrified because she was being operated on the next day. So I said some encouraging words to her, the way you would comfort any friend. It did her so much good that she asked me afterward if her doctor had sent me into her room. And I thought to myself, 'I know what doctor sent me.'"

The woman's roommate soon joined in on the conversation. To fully appreciate this scene, you have to know that Ms. Dawson is African-American and Christian and that the women with whom she bonded after eliciting the relaxation response were Caucasian and one was Jewish. And the story continues from there because not only did these three women go on to enjoy the results of the relaxation response, a nurse asked permission to wheel in an elderly Russian man who spoke very little English and who seemed very glum. However, the man did speak some Yiddish as did one of the women Ms. Dawson had met. So the four of them went on to converse about themselves, their hospitalizations, and the relaxation response.

At one point, Ms. Dawson remembers, the previously somber man's face was consumed with a smile, as he said how wonderful it felt to speak in Yiddish. He said he hadn't spoken it in years. Ms. Dawson remembers the hairs on the back of her neck creeping up when she heard him say it, and she made a mental snapshot of the four of them—so vastly different in culture, ethnicity, religion, and life experiences and yet sitting together in a hospital room, feeling for a few moments that they had everything in common.

"This is the rippling effect of the relaxation response—a feeling of being saturated with love," Ms. Dawson says. "That conglomeration of people and beliefs, that's what God wants to happen." Ms. Dawson is not the first of my patients to report this "rippling effect," a surge of good will and a feeling of commonalty with other people that makes them more respectful of others' religious beliefs. And I do think that by appreciating this physical bond of faith, this timeless, immutable fact of human life, people can be delivered from human-made divisions of racism, religious intolerance, and strife. I can imagine no greater health than this for humankind.

9. Believe in something good.

It is your destiny to believe in something good and something that lasts. But only you know what feels right for you. The pharmaceuticals and surgical procedures of modern medicine can do great things for you if your medical problems fall within their realms to heal. But much of the time, you have the power to heal yourself. And all of the time, you can enhance your health with remembered wellness.

Nevertheless, we should not expect to develop a faith in remembered wellness overnight. We've all been conditioned to believe in various sources of healing—in pills or doctors, in exercise or chiropractors, in herbs or prayer. It is not my intent in this book to undermine the things you believe have helped you heal. No matter how conscious you become of the fact that remembered wellness healed you, therapies that rely on remembered wellness such as herbs and acupuncture retain a subliminal power. Even though we do not necessarily need all the pills and procedures that conventional medicine and unconventional medicine give us, these medicinal symbols retain an aura of effectiveness and often appease our desire for action. While we must learn to use medicine more appropriately for the conditions it can help, and to wean ourselves from excessive spending on unnecessary therapies, we'll often need some catalysts for belief, even if belief is really the healer.

So remember the vigor from the time you felt healthiest in your life. Remember the blessing your mother said to you before you left for school, the smell of incense at church, or the tranquillity you felt picking up stones from the beach on Cape Cod. Remember the time the penicillin vanquished your ear infection, or the time the surgeon removed the splinter from deep in your foot and your pain immediately ceased. Remember how full-throated you sang in the choir or how long you stayed on the dance floor of a nightclub. Remember the doctor who really cared about you or the chaplain who prayed with you in the hospital. Remember the way you felt when you made love to your husband or wife, and the way you felt when your daughter or son was born.

Then let go, and believe. You've read all about your physiology, you've surrounded yourself with good caregivers who help you take a moderate, balanced approach to your health and health care. Now it's time to enjoy your endowment, this wiring for faith that makes the power of remembered wellness so enduring.

Believe in something good if you can. Or even better, believe in something better than anything you can fathom. Because for us mortals, this is very profound medicine.

A DISCLOSURE OF BELIEF

In the scientific world, it is well known that an investigator's beliefs and opinions can skew results if so permitted. This is what is called "bias." In what must seem entirely contradictory, given that this book is about the importance of one's personal beliefs, I am reluctant to share mine because of the training physicians receive, in which we must fiercely guard against bias—any influence that might contaminate our findings—and in which we are taught to shield our decisions from emotions.

But, just as researchers are required to disclose financial holdings that may be related to the experiments they conduct, I disclose my belief in God to allow you to judge for yourselves whether or not such a belief has affected my interpretation of the evidence. Disclosure is, I think, an important ingredient to look for in the books you read and in the medical practitioners you select.

I am astonished that my scientific studies have so conclusively shown that our bodies are wired to believe, that our bodies are nourished and healed by prayer and other exercises of belief. To me, this capability does not seem to be a fluke; our design does not seem haphazard. In the same way some physicists have found their scientific journeys inexorably leading to a conclusion of "deliberate supernatural design," my scientific studies have again and again returned to the potency of faith, so ingrained in the body that we cannot find a time in history when man and woman did not worship gods, pray, and entertain fervent beliefs. Whether God is conjured as an opiate for the masses, as Karl Marx suggested, or whether God created us to believe in an experience that is ever-soothing to us, the veracity of the experience of God is undeniable to me.

My reasoning and personal experience lead me to believe that there is a God. And yes, a thoughtful design must have been at work in the universe in which such definite patterns emerge, in which such incredible coincidences produced our world, and in which humans are wired to bear a physiologically healing faith. I believe in a scientifically describable biology and evolution and in a world that is, nonetheless, divinely influenced.

APPENDIX

RELAXATION AUDIO-
AND VIDEOTAPES

The following relaxation tapes are available through the Mind/Body Medical Institute, 110 Francis Street, Boston, MA 02215, (617) 632-9525. Each audiotape is $10; the video presentation is $35. Please make checks payable to the Mind/Body Medical Institute. Prices may change without notice. Proceeds benefit the programs of the Mind/Body Medical Institute.

Audiotapes

Basic Relaxation Exercise/Mindfulness Meditation
(female voice)
Side 1 (20 minutes) This side introduces a basic relaxation sequence to help you elicit the relaxation response, including some of the key elements such as breath awareness, body scan relaxation, and the use of a focus word. Specific instructions offered throughout the tape will aid your initial development in eliciting the relaxation response.
Side 2 (20 minutes) This side offers instruction on awareness, or "mindfulness," of sensations, thoughts, and sounds. It also introduces breath and awareness as "primary tools" that enable you to integrate the relaxation response into daily activities. This side has fewer instructions, allowing you to further develop your relaxation response techniques.

Basic Relaxation Response Exercise (male voice)
Side 1 (20 minutes) This tape is very similar to the aforementioned Basic Relaxation Exercise tape but features a male voice. It also introduces breath awareness and body scan relaxation.

Side 2 (45 minutes) Side 2 offers frequent pauses to encourage you to practice techniques that elicit the relaxation response.

Advanced Relaxation Response (female voice)
Side 1 (30 minutes) This side guides you through a body scan and relaxation, leading you into a relaxation response through awareness of your heart and repetition of your focus word. The tape has frequent pauses to encourage you to practice and develop ways of bringing forth the relaxation response on your own.
Side 2 (50 minutes) Side 2 reinforces basic skills and also guides you through a stretching routine and imagery for healing.

Guided Visualization with Ocean Sounds/Breath and Body Awareness (female voice)
Side 1 (24 minutes) Side 1 is a guided body scan relaxation. It incorporates guided visualization of a sandy ocean beach, enhanced by soothing ocean sounds in the background.
Side 2 (30 minutes) Side 2 leads you through a series of stretching exercises done in a sitting position. These stretches will encourage a peaceful state of relaxation, awareness, and the elicitation of the relaxation response. This side of the tape does not use ocean wave sounds.

Relaxation Exercise/Mountain Stream Mental Imagery (female voice)
Side 1 (20 minutes) This side gently guides you through a series of breathing techniques leading into body scan relaxation. Its purpose is to alleviate tension from each body part and allows you to practice breathing awareness. This side of the tape also includes a word focus exercise.
Side 2 (20 minutes) Side 2 offers you creative energy, acting as a tour guide on a walk through a forest to a mountain stream, allowing you to escape, to become aware of and focus on your senses.

Relaxation Response Extended Session/Beach Scene Mental Imagery (female voice)
Side 1 (40 minutes) Side 1 focuses on relaxation exercises, in-

---

cluding a long body scan relaxation to relieve tension from every part of your body. It then leads you through visualization of taking a warm, comfortable bath. The guidance in this tape is very specific, making it quite easy to follow. You may find this longer side useful during medical, surgical, or dental procedures.

Side 2 (20 minutes) Side 2 directs you through a series of breath and other relaxation exercises that elicit the relaxation response, followed by a guided imagery exercise of exploring a sandy beach on a magnificent summer day. (This tape features no ocean sounds.)

A Gift of Relaxation/Garden of Your Mind (female voice)
Side 1 (20 minutes) This side focuses on the basic steps of eliciting the relaxation response. You are quietly guided through a body scan relaxation exercise and some simple deep breathing techniques, which are intended to heighten your awareness and enable you to deepen your experience of the relaxation response. This tape ends with positive affirmations, encouraging you to feel good about yourself and to be proud of your experience.

Side 2 (20 minutes) This creative mental imagery exercise begins with body scan relaxation and breath awareness components and incorporates imagery of a lovely garden, one that you have visited in the past or one that you can create in your mind. The tape ends with positive self-statements and encouragement.

Tuning into Your Body, Tuning up Your Mind (female voice)
Side 1 (30 minutes) This side guides you through chair and standing exercises. The exercises emphasize releasing physical tension, loosening joints, and realigning posture. The practice session encourages elicitation of the relaxation response through mindfulness.

Side 2 (30 minutes) This side offers instruction in floor exercises found in *The Wellness Book*. It includes special instruction in diaphragmatic breathing and gives guidance for using your breath to enhance your exercise practice. This side ends with a deep relaxation. A diagram is included.

An Introduction to the Relaxation Response/A Special Time for You (female voice)

Side 1 (20 minutes) Side 1 introduces the elicitation of the relaxation response. It offers instruction in diaphragmatic breathing and the release of physical tension. The tape guides your practice by focusing on the breath, a word or phrase, and the creative imagination of a safe place. (This tape is suitable for people learning to elicit the relaxation response.)

Side 2 (20 minutes) This side gives gentle guidance in the practice of the relaxation response using imagery, body scan relaxation, and breath focus. The tape emphasizes the use of the breath and the practice of nonjudging awareness to decrease tension and to soothe physical discomfort.

Body Scan Relaxation with Ocean Sounds (female voice)

Side 1 (20 minutes) This side guides your elicitation of the relaxation response with a body scan and breathing focus, enhanced by ocean sounds in the background. This tape opens and closes with soothing piano music.

Side 2 (30 minutes) You listen to the soothing ocean sounds on side 2 to elicit the relaxation response without voice instruction.

Relaxation Response Exercises I and II (female voice)

Side 1 (20 minutes) This side introduces a basic relaxation sequence based on progressive muscle relaxation to help you elicit the relaxation response. Specific instructions throughout the tape aid in the initial development of your experience and the tape ends with a peaceful brief visualization.

Side 2 (14 minutes) This side guides you through a body scan and relaxation, leading you into the elicitation of the relaxation response and through an exercise of gently releasing tension throughout your body. The tape ends with a peaceful brief visualization.

Relaxation Response Exercise Tape (male voice)

Side 1 (31 minutes) This side offers instruction on how to elicit the relaxation response while exercising. This tape serves as a verbal guide to help you enhance mental health while improving your physical fitness.

Side 2 (31 minutes) This side has nondistracting music that fills the silence and is helpful once instruction featured on side 1 is no longer needed.

Rest in Gratitude/Healing Light (female voice)
Side 1 (19 minutes) This side uses guided imagery that invites you through a gentle body scan accompanied by soft music. You are asked to focus on and develop an awareness of various parts of your body. This is a very soothing and restful way to elicit the relaxation response and develop nonjudgmental, focused awareness.
Side 2 (19 minutes) This side uses breath awareness and ocean sounds and guides you to focus on a soothing, healing light. Rest and healing are emphasized. Ocean sounds are featured in the background.

Safe Place/Pain Visualization (female voice)
Side 1 (22 minutes) This side offers a guided meditation with progressive muscle relaxation and visualization of a safe place for patients with chronic pain. This tape will be helpful for those who might experience anxiety or feelings of vulnerability during the relaxation response process.
Side 2 (22 minutes) This side guides you through an advanced meditation with sweeps of progressive muscle relaxation and visualization of pain imagery. This is a potentially helpful exercise for pain control.

Basic Yoga Stretching Exercises/Stretching and Balancing Exercises (female voice)
Side 1 (20 minutes) Side 1 encourages you to focus on energizing your body. You are guided through a series of gentle stretches and relaxation exercises to reinforce diaphragmatic breathing. The moderate pace allows ample time to participate in the activities and to enhance your experience of the relaxation response. Side 1 ends in an exercise to elicit the relaxation response.
Side 2 (20 minutes) Side 2 encourages you to follow along in a gentle, slow-paced routine of stretching and movement awareness. Its purpose is to decrease muscular tension and elicit the relaxation response.

Body Scan, Breathing Techniques, and Autogenic Exercises
(male voice)
Side 1 (20 minutes) Body scan and breathing techniques combined with visual imagery.
Side 2 (30 minutes) Body scan, breathing techniques, and suggestions and imagery of warmth and heaviness in the body.

Relaxation Exercises for Students (female voices)
This tape is designed to guide students (ages nine through eighteen) in brief relaxation periods during a busy day. It is appropriate for use while sitting at a desk.
Side 1 (about 15 minutes) This side guides you through three short relaxation exercises including body scans, breath awareness, visualization (safe place), and music.
Side 2 (about 15 minutes) This side guides you through three more short relaxation exercises including body scans, breath awareness, visualization (mountain scenes), and music.

Videotape

An Introduction to the Mind/Body Medical Institute
This video presentation by Dr. Herbert Benson introduces the work of the Institute and the field of mind/body medicine, providing:

- a discussion of the physiology of the stress response and its counterpart, the relaxation response;
- a brief overview of the history of mind/body medicine; and
- a discussion of some aspects of mind/body medicine that are becoming more and more a part of mainstream medical practice.

REFERENCES

CHAPTER 1
A Search for Something That Lasts

Benson, H. *The Relaxation Response*. New York: William Morrow, 1975.

Benson, H., and M. D. Epstein. "The Placebo Effect—A Neglected Asset in the Care of Patients." *Journal of the American Medical Association* 232 (1975): 1225–27.

Benson, H. *The Mind/Body Effect*. New York: Simon & Schuster, 1979.

Benson, H., and D. P. McCallie, Jr. "Angina Pectoris and the Placebo Effect." *New England Journal of Medicine* 300 (1979): 1424–29.

Benson, H. *Beyond the Relaxation Response*. New York: Times Books, 1984.

Benson, H. *Your Maximum Mind*. New York: Times Books/Random House, 1987.

Benson, H., and E. M. Stuart. *The Wellness Book: A Comprehensive Guide to Maintaining Health and Treating Stress-Related Illness*. New York: Fireside, 1993.

Benson, H. "Commentary: Placebo Effect and Remembered Wellness." *Mind/Body Medicine* 1 (1995): 44–45.

Benson, H., and R. Friedman. "The Three-Legged Stool." *Mind/Body Medicine* 1 (1995): 1–2.

Benson, H., and R. Friedman. "Harnessing the Power of the Placebo Effect and Renaming It 'Remembered Wellness.'" *Annual Review of Medicine* 47 (1996): 193–99.

Cannon, W. B. "The Emergency Function of the Adrenal Medulla in Pain and the Major Emotions." *American Journal of Physiology* 33 (1914): 356–72.

Cannon, W. B. *Bodily Changes in Pain, Hunger, Fear and Rage:*

An Account of Recent Researches into the Function of Emotional Excitement. New York: Appleton, 1929.

CHAPTER 2
Remembered Wellness

Aldrich, C. K. "A Case of Recurrent Pseudocyesis." *Perspectives in Biology and Medicine* 16 (1972): 11–21.

Archer, T. P., and C. V. Leier. "Placebo Treatment in Congestive Heart Failure." *Cardiology* 81 (1992): 125–33.

Basedow, H. *The Australian Aboriginal.* Adelaide: F. W. Preece, 1925. As quoted in W. B. Cannon. " 'Voodoo' Death." *American Anthropologist* 44 (1942): 169–81.

Beecher, H. "The Powerful Placebo." *Journal of the American Medical Association* 159 (1955): 1602–6.

Benson, H., and M. D. Epstein. "The Placebo Effect—A Neglected Asset in the Care of Patients." *Journal of the American Medical Association* 232 (1975): 1225–27.

Benson, H. *The Mind/Body Effect.* New York: Simon & Schuster, 1979.

Benson, H., and D. P. McCallie, Jr. "Angina Pectoris and the Placebo Effect." *New England Journal of Medicine* 300 (1979): 1424–29.

Bivin, G. D., and M. P. Klinger. *Pseudocyesis.* Bloomington: Principia Press, 1937.

Cannon, W. B. " 'Voodoo' Death." *American Anthropologist* 44 (1942): 169–81.

Cannon, W. B. *The Way of an Investigator: A Scientist's Experiences in Medical Research.* New York: W.W. Norton, 1945.

Cebelin, M. S., and C. S. Hirsch. "Human Stress Cardiomyopathy: Myocardial Lesions in Victims of Homicidal Assaults Without Internal Injuries." *Human Pathology* 11 (1980): 123–32.

The Coronary Drug Project Research Group. "Influence of Adherence to Treatment and Response of Cholesterol on Mortality in the Coronary Drug Project." *New England Journal of Medicine* 303 (1980): 1038–41.

Egbert, L. D., G. E. Battit, C. E. Welch, and M. K. Bartlett. "Reduction of Postoperative Pain by Encouragement and Instruction of Patients." *New England Journal of Medicine* 270 (1964): 825–27.

Engel, G. "A Life Setting Conducive to Illness: The Giving-up–Given-up Complex." *Bulletin of the Menninger Clinic* 32 (1968): 355–65.

Engel, G. "Sudden and Rapid Death During Psychological Stress: Folklore or Folk Wisdom?" *Annals of Internal Medicine* 74 (1971): 771–82.

Fried, P. H., A. E. Rakoff, R. R. Schopbach, and A. J. Kaplan. "Pseudocyesis: A Psychosomatic Study in Gynecology." *Journal of the American Medical Association* 145 (1951): 1329–35.

Hashish, I., H. K. Hai, W. Harvey, C. Feinmann, and M. Harris. "Reduction of Postoperative Pain and Swelling by Ultrasound Treatment: A Placebo Effect." *Pain* 33 (1988): 303–11.

Hippocrates. "Precepts." As quoted in J. Bartlett. *Familiar Quotations.* Fourteenth Edition, E. M. Beck (ed.). Boston: Little, Brown, 1968.

Horwitz, R. I., C. M. Viscoli, L. Berkman, R. M. Donaldson, S. M. Horwitz, C. J. Murray, D. F. Ransohoff, and J. Sindelar. "Treatment Adherence and Risk of Death After a Myocardial Infarction." *Lancet* 336 (1990): 542–45.

Kannel, W. B., and P. D. Sorlie. "Remission of Clinical Angina Pectoris: The Framingham Study." *American Journal of Cardiology* 42 (1978): 119–23.

Kaplan, S., and S. Greenfield. "Enlarging Patient Responsibility." *Forum: Risk Management Foundation of the Harvard Medical Institutions* 14 (1993): 9–11.

Knight, J. A. "False Pregnancy in a Male." *Psychosomatic Medicine* 22 (1960): 260–66.

Kroger, W. S. *Psychosomatic Obstetrics, Gynecology and Endocrinology.* Springfield, IL: Charles C. Thomas, 1962.

Lesse, S. "Placebo Reactions in Psychotherapy." *Diseases of the Nervous System* 23 (1962): 313–19.

Menninger von Lerchenthal, E. "Death from Psychic Causes." *Bulletin of the Menninger Clinic* 12 (1948): 31–36.

Murray, J. L., and G. E. Abraham. "Pseudocyesis: A Review." *Obstetrics and Gynecology* 51 (1978): 627–31.

The Oxford English Dictionary. J. A. Murray (ed.). Oxford: Clarendon Press, 1909.

Pickering, T. G. "Blood Pressure Variability and Ambulatory Monitoring." *Current Opinion in Nephrology and Hypertension* 2 (1993): 380–85.

Pogge, R. "The Toxic Placebo." *Medical Times* 91 (1963): 773–78.

Roberts, A. H., D. G. Kewman, L. Mercier, and M. Hovell. "The Power of Nonspecific Effects in Healing: Implications for Psychosocial and Biological Treatments." *Clinical Psychology Review* 13 (1993): 375–91.

Saul, L. J. "Sudden Death at Impasse." *Psychoanalytic Forum* 1 (1966): 88–89.

Thomas, K. B. "General Practice Consultations: Is There Any Point in Being Positive?" *British Medical Journal Clinical Research* 294 (1987): 1200–2.

Tilley, B. C., G. S. Alarcon, S. P. Heyse, D. E. Trentham, R. Neuner, D. A. Kaplan, D. O. Clegg, J. C. Leisen, L. Buckley, S. M. Cooper, H. Duncan, S. R. Pillemer, M. Tuttleman, and S. E. Fowler. "Minocycline in Rheumatoid Arthritis: A 48-week, Double-Blind, Placebo-Controlled Trial." *Annals of Internal Medicine* 122 (1995): 81–89.

Traut, E. F., and E. W. Passarelli. "Placebos in the Treatment of Rheumatoid Arthritis and Other Rheumatic Conditions." *Annals of the Rheumatic Diseases* 16 (1957): 18–22.

Turner, J. A., R. A. Deyo, J. D. Loeser, M. Von Korff, and W. E. Fordyce. "The Importance of Placebo Effects in Pain Treatment and Research." *Journal of the American Medical Association* 271 (1994): 1609–14.

Wolf, S. "Effects of Suggestion and Conditioning on the Action of Chemical Agents in Human Subjects: The Pharmacology of Placebos." *Journal of Clinical Investigation* 29 (1950): 100–9.

CHAPTER 3
The Nature of Belief

Adams, J. As quoted in J. Bartlett. *Familiar Quotations.* Fourteenth Edition, E. M. Beck (ed.). Boston: Little, Brown, 1968.

Bates, M. S., W. T. Edwards, and K. O. Anderson. "Ethnocultural Influences on Variation in Chronic Pain Perception." *Pain* 52 (1993): 101–12.

Blackwell, B., S. S. Bloomfield, and C. R. Buncher. "Demonstration to Medical Students of Placebo Responses and Non-Drug Factors." *Lancet* 1 (1972): 1279–82.

Buckalew, L. W., and K. E. Coffield. "An Investigation of Drug Expectancy as a Function of Capsule Color and Size and Preparation Form." *Journal of Clinical Psychopharmacology* 2 (1982): 245–48.

Butler, C., and A. Steptoe. "Placebo Responses: An Experimental Study of Psychophysiological Processes in Asthmatic Volunteers." *British Journal of Clinical Psychology* 25 (1986): 173–83.

Cummings, N. A., and G. R. VandenBos. "The Twenty Years Kaiser-Permanente Experience with Psychotherapy and Medical Utilization: Implications for National Health Policy and National Health Insurance." *Health Policy Quarterly* 1 (1981): 159–75.

Daniels, A. M., and R. Sallie. "Headache, Lumbar Puncture and Expectation." *Lancet* 1 (1981): 1003.

Eisenberg, D. M., R. C. Kessler, C. Foster, F. E. Norlock, D. R. Calkins, and T. L. Delbanco. "Unconventional Medicine in the United States: Prevalence, Costs and Patterns of Use." *New England Journal of Medicine* 328 (1993): 246–52.

Franco, K., N. Campbell, M. Tamburrino, S. Jurs, J. Pentz, and C. Evans. "Anniversary Reactions and Due Date Responses Following Abortion." *Psychotherapy and Psychosomatics* 52 (1989): 151–54.

Fry, J. *Profiles of Disease: A Study in the Natural History of Common Diseases.* Edinburgh: E. and S. Livingstone, 1966.

Huskisson, E. C. "Simple Analgesics for Arthritis." *British Medical Journal* 4 (1974): 196–200.

Ikemi, Y., and S. Nakagawa. "A Psychosomatic Study of Contagious Dermatitis." *Kyoshu Journal of Medical Science* 13 (1962): 335–50.

Ingelfinger, F. J. "Medicine: Meritorious or Meretricious." *Science* 200 (1978): 942–46.

Jefferson, T. As quoted in J. Bartlett. *Familiar Quotations.* Fourteenth Edition, E. M. Beck (ed.). Boston: Little, Brown, 1968.

Kristof, N. D. "Kobe's Survivors Try to Adjust: Hand-Wringing, Relief, Laughter." *New York Times*, January 22, 1995, p. 1.

Kroenke, K., and A. D. Mangelsdorff. "Common Symptoms in Ambulatory Care: Incidence, Evaluation, Therapy and Outcome." *American Journal of Medicine* 86 (1989): 262–66.

Lucchelli, P. E., A. D. Cattaneo, and J. Zattoni. "Effect of Capsule Colour and Order of Administration of Hypnotic Treatments." *European Journal of Clinical Pharmacology* 13 (1978): 153–55.

Phillips, D. P., C. A. Van Voorhees, and T. E. Ruth. "The Birthday: Lifeline or Deadline?" *Psychosomatic Medicine* 54 (1992): 532–42.

Riley, J. F., D. K. Ahern, and M. J. Follick. "Chronic Pain and Functional Impairment: Assessing Beliefs About Their Relationship." *Archives of Physical Medicine and Rehabilitation* 69 (1988): 579–82.

Roethlisberger, F. J., and W. J. Dickson. *Management and the Worker: An Account of a Research Program Conducted by the Western Electric Company, Hawthorne Works, Chicago.* Cambridge, MA: Harvard University Press, 1949.

Sobel, D. "All in Your Head." *Mental Medicine Update* 3 (1995).

Sternbach, R. A., and B. Tursky. "Ethnic Differences Among Housewives in Psychophysical and Skin Potential Responses to Electric Shock." *Psychophysiology* 1 (1965): 241–46.

Weisman, A. D., and T. P. Hackett. "Predilection to Death: Death and Dying as a Psychiatric Problem." *Psychosomatic Medicine* 23 (1961): 232–56.

Zborowski, M. "Cultural Components in Responses to Pain." *Journal of Social Issues* 8 (1952): 16–30.

CHAPTER 4
The Brain's Prerogative

Adler, S. R. "Ethnomedical Pathogenesis and Hmong Immigrants' Sudden Nocturnal Deaths." *Culture, Medicine and Psychiatry* 18 (1994): 23–59.

Bargh, J. As quoted in D. Goleman. "Brain May Tag All Perceptions with a Value." *New York Times*, August 8, 1995, p. C1.

Barinaga, M. "Watching the Brain Remake Itself." *Science* 266 (1994): 1475–76.

Churchland, P. M. *The Engine of Reason, The Seat of the Soul: A Philosophical Journey into the Brain.* Cambridge, MA: A Bradford Book, MIT Press, 1995.

Cytowic, R. E. *The Man Who Tasted Shapes: A Bizarre Medical Mystery Offers Revolutionary Insights into Emotions, Reasoning and Consciousness.* New York: G. P. Putnam, 1993.

Damasio, A. *Descartes' Error: Emotion, Reason and the Human Brain.* New York: Grosset/Putnam, 1994.

Damasio, H., T. J. Grabowski, A. Damasio, D. Tranel, L. Boles-Ponto, G. L. Watkins, and R. D. Hichwa. "Visual Recall with Eyes Closed and Covered Activates Early Visual Cortices." *Abstracts Society for Neuroscience* 19 (1993): 1603.

De Cuevas, J. "Mind, Brain and Behavior." *Harvard Magazine* (1994): 36–43.

George, M. S., T. A. Ketter, P. I. Parekh, B. Horwitz, P. Herscovitch, and R. M. Post. "Brain Activity During Transient Sadness and Happiness in Healthy Women." *American Journal of Psychiatry* 152 (1995): 341–51.

Gibson, E. J., and R. Walk. "The 'Visual Cliff.' " *Scientific American* 202 (1960): 64–71.

Goleman, D. "The Brain Manages Happiness and Sadness in Different Centers." *New York Times*, March 28, 1995, pp. C8–C9.

Gur, R. C., L. H. Mozley, P. D. Mozley, S. M. Resnick, J. S. Karp,

A. Alavi, S. E. Arnold, and R. E. Gur. "Sex Differences in Regional Cerebral Glucose Metabolism During a Resting State." *Science* 267 (1995): 528–31.

Hess, W. R., and M. Brugger. "Das Subkortikzle Zentrum der Affektiven Abwehrreaktion." *Helvetica Physiologica et Pharmacologica Acta* 1 (1943): 33–52.

Hess, W. R. *The Functional Organization of the Diencephalon.* New York: Grune and Stratton, 1957.

James, W. "What Psychical Research Has Accomplished." As quoted in R. Moore (ed.). *In Search of White Crows: Spiritualism, Parapsychology, and American Culture.* New York: Oxford University Press, 1977.

Karni, A. "When Practice Makes Perfect." *Lancet* 345 (1995): 395.

Katz, J., and R. Melzack. "Pain 'Memories' in Phantom Limbs: Review and Clinical Observations." *Pain* 43 (1990): 319–36.

Kosslyn, S., N. M. Alpert, W. L. Thompson, V. Maljkovic, S. B. Weise, C. F. Chabris, S. E. Hamilton, S. L. Rauch, and F. S. Buonanno. "Visual Mental Imagery Activates Topographically Organized Visual Cortex: PET Investigations." *Journal of Cognitive Neuroscience* 5 (1993): 263–87.

Kosslyn, S. *Image and Brain: The Resolution of the Imagery Debate.* Cambridge, MA: MIT Press, 1994.

Melzack, R. "Phantom Limbs." *Scientific American* 266 (1992): 120–26.

Miyashita, Y. "How the Brain Creates Imagery: Projection to Primary Visual Cortex." *Science* 268 (1995): 1719–20.

Murray, E. J., and F. Foote. "The Origins of Fear of Snakes." *Behaviour Research and Therapy* 17 (1979): 489–93.

Oppenheimer, S. M., J. X. Wilson, C. Guirauden, and D. F. Cechetto. "Insular Cortex Stimulation Produces Lethal Cardiac Arrhythmias: A Mechanism of Sudden Death?" *Brain Research* 550 (1991): 115–21.

Oppenheimer, S. M. "The Broken Heart: Noninvasive Measurement of Cardiac Autonomic Tone." *Postgraduate Medical Journal* 68 (1992): 939–41.

Oppenheimer, S. M., A. Gelb, J. P. Girvin, and V. C. Hachinski. "Cardiovascular Effects of Human Insular Cortex Stimulation." *Neurology* 42 (1992): 1727–32.

Pellegrino, C. *Return to Sodom and Gomorrah: Bible Stories from Archaeologists*. New York: Random House, 1994.

Rothbaum, B. As quoted in "Virtual Therapy for Phobias." *Science* 268 (1995): 209.

Walk, R., and E. J. Gibson. "A Comparative and Analytical Study of Visual Depth Perception." *Psychological Monographs* 75 (1961): 15.

CHAPTER 5
Medicine's Spiritual Crisis

Ackerknecht, E. H. *Medicine and Ethnology*. Baltimore: Johns Hopkins Press, 1971.

Altman, L. K. "Medical Errors Bring Calls for Change." *New York Times*, July 18, 1995.

Angell, M., and J. Kassirer. "What Should the Public Believe?" *New England Journal of Medicine* 331 (1994): 189–90.

Annas, G. J., and F. H. Miller. "The Empire of Death: How Culture and Economics Affect Informed Consent in the U.S., the U.K. and Japan." *American Journal of Law and Medicine* 20 (1994): 357–94.

Barzini, L. *The Europeans*. New York: Simon & Schuster, 1983.

Blumenthal, D. "Making Medical Errors into 'Medical Treasures.' " *Journal of the American Medical Association* 272 (1994): 1867–68.

Cabot, R. C. "The Use of Truth and Falsehood in Medicine." *Connecticut Medicine* 42 (1978): 189–94.

Cohen, M. As quoted in "Never Mind Ebola, We Have Defiant Bugs." *San Diego Union-Tribune*, May 17, 1995, p. A-18.

Eisenberg, D. M., R. C. Kessler, C. Foster, F. E. Norlock, D. R. Calkins, and T. L. Delbanco. "Unconventional Medicine in the United States: Prevalence, Costs and Patterns of Use." *New England Journal of Medicine* 328 (1993): 246–52.

Fein, E. B. "Competing Hospitals Are Nicer to Patients." *New York Times*, July 24, 1995.

Flexner, A. *Medical Education in the United States and Canada: A Report to the Carnegie Foundation for the Advancement of*

Teaching. New York: Carnegie Foundation for the Advancement of Teaching, 1910.

Gelfand, M. *Medicine and Custom in Africa.* Edinburgh: E. and S. Livingstone, 1964.

Gelfand, M. *Witch Doctor: The Traditional Medicine Man of Rhodesia.* London: Harvill Press, 1964.

Gelfand, M. *The African Witch, with Particular Reference to Witchcraft Beliefs and Practice Among the Shona of Rhodesia.* London: E. and S. Livingstone, 1967.

Gillon, R. " 'Primum Non Nocere' and the Principle of Non-Malfeasance." *British Medical Journal Clinical Research Ed.* 291 (1985): 130–31.

Golub, E. S. *The Limits of Medicine: How Science Shapes Our Hope for the Cure.* New York: Times Books, 1994.

Gregg, J. "Commerce of the Prairies, or The Journal of a Sante Fe Trader." In *Early Western Travels.* R. G. Thwaites (ed.). 1905. As quoted in V. J. Vogel. *American Indian Medicine.* Norman: University of Oklahoma Press, 1970.

Hand, W. D. *Magical Medicine: The Folkloric Component of Medicine in the Folk Belief, Custom and Ritual of the Peoples of Europe and America.* Berkeley: University of California Press, 1980.

Hofling, C. K. "The Place of Placebos in Medical Practice." *G P* XI (1955): 103–7.

Holden, C. " 'Iceman' Markings Seen as Medical Tattoos." *Science* 268 (1995): 33.

Holmes, O. W. *The Writings of Oliver Wendell Holmes.* Vol. 9, Medical Essays. Cambridge, MA: Riverside Press, 1891.

Lazear-Asher, B. "Spa Wars." *Self* (July 1995): 42–44.

Leape, L. L. "Error in Medicine." *Journal of the American Medical Association* 272 (1994): 1851–57.

Leape, L. L., D. W. Bates, D. J. Cullen, J. Cooper, H. J. Demonaco, T. Gallivan, R. Hallisey, J. Ives, N. Laird, G. Laffel, R. Nemeskal, L. A. Petersen, K. Porter, D. Servi, B. F. Shea, S. D. Small, B. J. Sweitzer, B. T. Thompson, and M. Vander Vliet. "Systems Analysis of Adverse Drug Events." *Journal of the American Medical Association* 274 (1995): 35–43.

The Macmillan Dictionary of Quotations. New York: Macmillan, 1989.

Myers, S. S., and H. Benson. "Psychological Factors in Healing: A New Perspective on an Old Debate." *Behavioral Medicine* 18 (1992): 5–11.

Nuland, S. B. "Medical Fads: Bran, Midwives and Leeches." *New York Times,* June 25, 1995, p. E16.

Rosenberg, C. "The Therapeutic Revolution." In *Sickness and Health in America: Readings in the History of Medicine and Public Health.* J. Leavitt and R. Numbers (eds.). 2nd ed. Madison: University of Wisconsin Press, 1985.

Shapiro, A. K. "A Contribution to a History of the Placebo Effect." *Behavior Science Notes* 5 (1960): 109–35.

Shapiro, A. K. "Factors Contributing to the Placebo Effect." *American Journal of Psychotherapy* 18 (1961): 73–88.

Shapiro, A. K. "Semantics of the Placebo." *Psychiatric Quarterly* 42 (1968): 653–95.

Shapiro, A. K. "Placebo Effects in Medicine, Psychotherapy and Psychoanalysis." In *Handbook of Psychotherapy and Behavior Change: An Empirical Analysis.* A. E. Bergin and S. L. Garfield (eds.). New York: Wiley, 1971, pp. 439–73.

Shapiro, A. K., and E. L. Struening. "A Comparison of the Attitudes of a Sample of Physicians About the Effectiveness of Their Treatment and the Treatment of Other Physicians." *Journal of Psychiatric Research* 10 (1974): 217–29.

Shapiro, A. K., and L. Morris. "The Placebo Effect in Medical and Psychological Therapies." In *Handbook of Psychotherapy and Behavior Change: An Empirical Analysis.* S. L. Garfield and A. E. Bergin (eds.). 2nd ed. New York: Wiley, 1978, pp. 477–536.

Sontag, S. *Illness As Metaphor.* New York: Farrar, Straus & Giroux, 1978.

Taubes, G. "Epidemiology Faces Its Limits: The Search for Subtle Links Between Diet, Lifestyle, or Environmental Factors and Disease Is an Unending Source of Fear—But Often Yields Little Certainty." *Science* 269 (1995): 164–69.

U.S. Department of Health and Human Services. *Health United States 1993.* Pub. No. (PHS) 94-1232. Hyattsville, MD: Public Health Service, 1994.

Updike, J. *Rabbit at Rest.* New York: Knopf, 1990.

CHAPTER 6
The Relaxation Response

Beary, J. F., and H. Benson. "A Simple Psychophysiologic Technique Which Elicits the Hypometabolic Changes of the Relaxation Response." *Psychosomatic Medicine* 36 (1974): 115–20.

Benson, H., B. P. Malvea, and J. R. Graham. "Physiologic Correlates of Meditation and Their Clinical Effects in Headache: An Ongoing Investigation." *Headache* 13 (1973): 23–24.

Benson, H., J. F. Beary, and M. P. Carol. "The Relaxation Response." *Psychiatry* 37 (1974): 37–46.

Benson, H., H. P. Klemchuk, and J. R. Graham. "The Usefulness of the Relaxation Response in the Therapy of Headache." *Headache* 14 (1974): 49–52.

Benson, H., B. A. Rosner, B. R. Marzetta, and H. P. Klemchuk. "Decreased Blood Pressure in Borderline Hypertensive Subjects Who Practiced Meditation." *Journal of Chronic Diseases* 27 (1974): 163–69.

Benson, H. *The Relaxation Response.* New York: William Morrow, 1975.

Benson, H., S. Alexander, and C. L. Feldman. "Decreased Premature Ventricular Contractions Through Use of the Relaxation Response in Patients with Stable Ischaemic Heart-Disease." *Lancet* 2 (1975): 380–82.

Benson, H., T. Dryer, and L. H. Hartley. "Decreased VO2 Consumption During Exercise with Elicitation of the Relaxation Response." *Journal of Human Stress* 4 (1978): 38–42.

Benson, H., F. H. Frankel, R. Apfel, M. D. Daniels, H. E. Schniewind, J. C. Nemiah, P. E. Sifneos, K. D. Crassweller, M. M. Greenwood, J. B. Kotch, P. A. Arns, and B. Rosner. "Treatment of Anxiety: A Comparison of the Usefulness of Self-Hypnosis and a Meditational Relaxation Technique." *Psychotherapy and Psychosomatics* 30 (1978): 229–42.

Benson, H., P. A. Arns, and J. W. Hoffman. "The Relaxation

Response and Hypnosis." *International Journal of Clinical and Experimental Hypnosis* 29 (1981): 259–70.

Benson, H. "The Relaxation Response: Its Subjective and Objective Historical Precedents and Physiology." *TINS* 6 (1983): 281–84.

Benson, H. *Beyond the Relaxation Response.* New York: Times Books, 1984.

Benson, H. *Your Maximum Mind.* New York: Times Books/Random House, 1987.

Benson, H. and E. M. Stuart. *The Wellness Book: A Comprehensive Guide to Maintaining Health and Treating Stress-Related Illness.* New York: Fireside, 1993.

Benson, H., A. Kornhaber, C. Kornhaber, M. N. LeChanu, P. C. Zuttermeister, P. Myers, and R. Friedman. "Increases in Positive Psychological Characteristics with a New Relaxation-Response Curriculum in High School Students." *Journal for Research and Development in Education* 27 (1994): 226–31.

Carrington, P., G. H. Collings, H. Benson, H. Robinson, L. W. Wood, P. M. Lehrer, R. L. Woolfolk, and J. W. Cole. "The Use of Meditation–Relaxation Techniques for the Management of Stress in a Working Population." *Journal of Occupational Medicine* 22 (1980): 221–31.

Caudill, M., R. Schnable, P. C. Zuttermeister, H. Benson, and R. Friedman. "Decreased Clinic Utilization by Chronic Pain Patients: Response to Behavioral Medicine Intervention." *Clinical Journal of Pain* 7 (1991): 305–10.

Caudill, M. *Managing Pain Before It Manages You.* New York: Guilford, 1994.

Cummings, N. A., and G. R. VandenBos. "The Twenty Years Kaiser-Permanente Experience with Psychotherapy and Medical Utilization: Implications for National Health Policy and National Health Insurance." *Health Policy Quarterly* 1 (1981): 159–75.

Cytowic, R. E. *The Man Who Tasted Shapes: A Bizarre Medical Mystery Offers Revolutionary Insights into Emotions, Reasoning and Consciousness.* New York: G. P. Putnam, 1993.

Domar, A. D., M. M. Seibel, and H. Benson. "The Mind/Body

Program for Infertility: A New Behavioral Treatment Approach for Women with Infertility." *Fertility and Sterility* 53 (1990): 246–49.

Domar, A. D., P. C. Zuttermeister, M. Seibel, and H. Benson. "Psychological Improvement in Infertile Women After Behavioral Treatment: A Replication." *Fertility and Sterility* 58 (1992): 144–47.

Fentress, D. W., B. J. Masek, J. E. Mehegan, and H. Benson. "Biofeedback and Relaxation-Response Training in the Treatment of Pediatric Migraine." *Developmental Medicine and Child Neurology* 28 (1986): 139–46.

Goodale, I. L., A. D. Domar, and H. Benson. "Alleviation of Premenstrual Syndrome Symptoms with the Relaxation Response." *Obstetrics and Gynecology* 75 (1990): 649–55.

Hellman, C. J., M. Budd, J. Borysenko, D. C. McClelland, and H. Benson. "A Study of the Effectiveness of Two Group Behavioral Medicine Interventions for Patients with Psychosomatic Complaints." *Behavioral Medicine* 16 (1990): 165–73.

Hoffman, J. W., H. Benson, P. A. Arns, G. L. Stainbrook, G. L. Landsberg, J. B. Young, and A. Gill. "Reduced Sympathetic Nervous System Responsivity Associated with the Relaxation Response." *Science* 215 (1982): 190–92.

Huang, Guozhi. "Physiological Effects During Relaxation Qigong Exercise." *Psychosomatic Medicine* 53 (1991): 228.

Jacobs, G. D., H. Benson, and R. Friedman. "Home-Based Central Nervous System Assessment of a Multifactor Behavioral Intervention for Chronic Sleep-Onset Insomnia." *Behavior Therapy* 24 (1993): 159–74.

Jacobs, G. D., P. A. Rosenberg, R. Friedman, J. Matheson, G. M. Peavy, A. D. Domar, and H. Benson. "Multifactor Behavioral Treatment of Chronic Sleep-Onset Insomnia Using Stimulus Control and the Relaxation Response: A Preliminary Study." *Behavior Modification* 17 (1993): 498–509.

Leserman, J., E. Stuart, M. E. Mamish, and H. Benson. "The Efficacy of the Relaxation Response in Preparing for Cardiac Surgery." *Behavioral Medicine* 15 (1989): 111–17.

Leserman, J., E. Stuart, M.E. Mamish, J. Deckro, R. J. Beckam, R. Friedman, and H. Benson. "Nonpharmacologic Intervention for Hypertension: Long-Term Follow-up." *Journal of Cardiopulmonary Rehabilitation* 9 (1989): 316–24.

Linden, W., and L. Chambers. "Clinical Effectiveness of Non-Drug Treatment for Hypertension: A Meta-Analysis." *Annals of Behavioral Medicine* 16 (1994): 35–45.

Mandle, C. L., A. D. Domar, D. P. Harrington, J. Leserman, E. M. Bozadjian, R. Friedman, and H. Benson. "Relaxation Response in Femoral Angiography." *Radiology* 174 (1990): 737–39.

Mundy, L. *Prayer Walking*. T G. Harris (ed.). St. Meinrad, IN: Abbey Press, 1994.

Peters, R. K., H. Benson, and J. M. Peters. "Daily Relaxation Response Breaks in a Working Population: II. Effects on Blood Pressure." *American Journal of Public Health* 67 (1977): 954–59.

Peters, R. K., H. Benson, and D. Porter. "Daily Relaxation Response Breaks in a Working Population: I. Effects on Self-Reported Measures of Health, Performance and Well-being." *American Journal of Public Health* 67 (1977): 946–53.

Stuart, E., M. Caudill, J. Leserman, C. Dorrington, R. Friedman, and H. Benson. "Nonpharmacologic Treatment of Hypertension: A Multiple-Risk-Factor Approach." *Journal of Cardiovascular Nursing* 1 (1987): 1–14.

Wallace, R. K., H. Benson, and A. F. Wilson. "A Wakeful Hypometabolic Physiologic State." *American Journal of Physiology* 221 (1971): 795–99.

Wallace, R. K., and H. Benson. "The Physiology of Meditation." *Scientific American* 226 (1972): 369–79.

Wang, Y., D. Brown, C. B. Ebbeling, L. Fortlage, J. Samuels, L. Ahlquist, A. Ward, J. Rippe, and H. Benson. "Acute Psychological Response Following Exercise and Exercise Plus Relaxation." *American College of Sports Medicine* (1992).

CHAPTER 7
The Faith Factor
and the Spiritual Experience

Armstrong, K. *A History of God: The 4,000-Year Quest of Judaism, Christianity and Islam.* New York: Knopf, 1993.

Benson, H., J. F. Beary, and M. P. Carol. "The Relaxation Response." *Psychiatry* 37 (1974): 37–46.

Benson, H. *The Relaxation Response.* New York: William Morrow, 1975.

Benson, H. "Body Temperature Changes During the Practice of g Tum-mo Yoga." *Nature* 298 (1982): 402.

Benson, H., J. W. Lehmann, M. S. Malhotra, R. F. Goldman, J. Hopkins, and M. D. Epstein. "Body Temperature Changes During the Practice of g Tum-mo (Heat) Yoga." *Nature* 295 (1982): 234–36.

Benson, H. *Beyond the Relaxation Response.* New York: Times Books, 1984.

Benson, H. *Your Maximum Mind.* New York: Times Books/ Random House, 1987.

Benson, H., M. S. Malhotra, R. F. Goldman, G. D. Jacobs, and P. J. Hopkins. "Three Case Reports of the Metabolic and Electroencephalographic Changes During Advanced Buddhist Meditation Techniques." *Behavioral Medicine* 16 (1990): 90–95.

Blackmore, S. *Dying to Live: Near-Death Experiences.* Buffalo, New York: Prometheus Books, 1993.

Dean, S. R. "Metapsychiatry: The Confluence of Psychiatry and Mysticism." In *Psychiatry and Mysticism.* S. R. Dean (ed.). Chicago: Nelson-Hall, 1975.

Frank, A. *The Diary of a Young Girl.* New York: Modern Library, 1952.

Harpur, T. *The Uncommon Touch: An Investigation of Spiritual Healing.* Toronto: McLelland & Stewart, 1994.

Holy Qur'an. M. H. Shakir (ed.). New York: Tahrike Tarsile Qur'an, 1982.

The Holy Bible: Old and New Testaments in the King James Version. Nashville, TN: Nelson, 1983.

Huang Guozhi. "Physiological Effects During Relaxation Qigong Exercise." *Psychosomatic Medicine* 53 (1991): 228.

James, W. *The Varieties of Religious Experience.* Cambridge, MA: Harvard University Press, 1985.

Johnson, R. S. "Lloyd Advances to Open Semifinal." *New York Times*, September 4, 1986.

Kantrowitz, B., P. King, D. Rosenberg, K. Springen, P. Wingert, T. Namuth, and T. T. Gegax. "In Search of the Sacred." *Newsweek* (November 28, 1994): 52–62.

Kass, J. D., R. Friedman, J. Leserman, P. C. Zuttermeister, and H. Benson. "Health Outcomes and a New Index of Spiritual Experience." *Journal for the Scientific Study of Religion* 30 (1991): 203–11.

Levin, J. S. "Religion and Health: Is There an Association, Is It Valid, and Is It Causal?" *Social Science and Medicine* 38 (1994): 1475–82.

McKee, D., and J. Chappel. "Spirituality and Medical Practice." *Journal of Family Practice* 35 (1992): 201, 205–8.

Noble, H. B. " 'Zone' Is Winning Territory." *New York Times*, September 5, 1986.

Osler, W. "The Faith That Heals." *British Medical Journal* 18 (1910): 1470–72.

CHAPTER 8

Faith Heals

Amoateng, A. Y., and S. J. Bahr. "Religion, Family and Adolescent Drug Use." *Sociological Perspectives* 29 (1986): 53–76.

Armstrong, K. *A History of God: The 4,000-Year Quest of Judaism, Christianity and Islam.* New York: Knopf, 1993.

Benor, D. J. "Survey of Spiritual Healing Research." *Complementary Medical Research* 4 (1990): 9–33.

Berkel, J., and F. de Waard. "Mortality Pattern and Life Expectancy of Seventh-Day Adventists in the Netherlands." *International Journal of Epidemiology* 12 (1983): 455–59.

Berkman, L. F., and S. L. Syme. "Social Networks, Host Resistance, and Mortality: A Nine-Year Follow-up Study of

Alameda County Residents." *American Journal of Epidemi-ology* 109 (1979): 186–204.

Beutler, J. J., J. T. Attevelt, S. A. Schouten, J. A. Faber, E. J. Dorhout Mees, and G. G. Geijskes. "Paranormal Healing and Hypertension." *British Medical Journal Clinical Research Ed.* 296 (1988): 1491–94.

Byrd, R. C. "Positive Therapeutic Effects of Intercessory Prayer in a Coronary Care Unit Population." *Southern Medical Journal* 81 (1988): 826–29.

Carrington, P., G. H. Collings, H. Benson, H. Robinson, L. W. Wood, P. M. Lehrer, R. L. Woolfolk, and J. W. Cole. "The Use of Meditation–Relaxation Techniques for the Management of Stress in a Working Population." *Journal of Occupational Medicine* 22 (1980): 221–31.

Dossey, L. *Healing Words: The Power of Prayer and the Practice of Medicine.* New York: HarperCollins, 1993.

Enstrom, J. E. "Health Practices and Cancer Mortality Among Active California Mormons." *Journal of the National Cancer Institute* 81 (1989): 1807–14.

Gallup, G. H., Jr., and S. Jones. *100 Questions and Answers: Religion in America.* Princeton: Princeton Religion Research Center, 1989.

Gallup, G. H., Jr. *Religion in America: 1990.* Princeton: Princeton Religion Research Center, 1990.

Gilk, D. C. "The Redefinition of the Situation: The Social Construction of Spiritual Healing Experiences." *Sociology of Health and Illness* 12 (1990): 151–68.

Heidt, P. R. "Effect of Therapeutic Touch on Anxiety Level of Hospitalized Patients." *Nursing Research* 30 (1981): 32–37.

The Holy Bible: Old and New Testaments in the King James Version. Nashville, TN: Nelson, 1983.

House, J. S., C. Robbins, and H. L. Metzner. "The Association of Social Relationships and Activities with Mortality: Prospective Evidence from the Tecumseh Community Health Study." *American Journal of Epidemiology* 116 (1982): 123–40.

Jensen, O. M. "Cancer Risk Among Danish Male Seventh-Day Adventists and Other Temperance Society Members." *Journal of the National Cancer Institute* 70 (1983): 1011–14.

Johnson, D. M., J. S. Williams, and D. G. Bromley. "Religion, Health and Healing: Findings from a Southern City." *Sociological Analysis* 46 (1986): 66–73.

Keller, E., and V. M. Bzdek. "Effects of Therapeutic Touch on Tension Headache Pain." *Nursing Research* 35 (1986): 101–6.

Larson, D. B. *The Faith Factor: An Annotated Bibliography of Systematic Reviews and Clinical Research on Spiritual Subjects.* Vol 2. John Templeton Foundation, 1993.

Levin, J. S., and P. L. Schiller. "Is There a Religious Factor in Health?" *Journal of Religion and Health* 26 (1987): 9–36.

Levin, J. S., and H. Y. Vanderpool. "Is Frequent Religious Attendance *Really* Conducive to Better Health? Toward an Epidemiology of Religion." *Social Science and Medicine* 24 (1987): 589–600.

Levin, J. S. "Religion and Health: Is There an Association, Is It Valid, and Is It Causal?" *Social Science and Medicine* 38 (1994): 1475–82.

Luks, A. *The Healing Power of Doing Good.* New York: Ballantine, 1993.

Luther, M. *Table Talk.* As quoted in J. Bartlett. *Familiar Quotations.* Fourteenth Edition, E. M. Beck (ed.). Boston: Little, Brown, 1968, p. 352.

Mason, R. C., Jr., G. Clark, R. B. Reeves, Jr., and S. B. Wagner. "Acceptance and Healing." *Journal of Religion and Health* 8 (1969): 123.

Matthews, D. A., D. B. Larson, and C. P. Barry. *The Faith Factor: An Annotated Bibliography of Clinical Research on Spiritual Subjects.* Vol 1. John Templeton Foundation, 1993.

Meehan, T. C. "Therapeutic Touch and Postoperative Pain: A Rogerian Research Study." *Nursing Science Quarterly* 6 (1993): 69–78.

Orr, R. D., and G. Isaac. "Religious Variables Are Infrequently Reported in Clinical Research." *Family Medicine* 24 (1992): 602–6.

Oxman, T. E., D. H. Freeman, Jr., and E. D. Manheimer. "Lack of Social Participation or Religious Strength and Comfort As Risk Factors for Death After Cardiac Surgery in the Elderly." *Psychosomatic Medicine* 57 (1995): 5–15.

Pressman, P., J. S. Lyons, D. B. Larson, and J. J. Strain. "Religious Belief, Depression, and Ambulation Status in Elderly Women with Broken Hips." *American Journal of Psychiatry* 147 (1990): 758–60.

Schiller, P. L., and J. S. Levin. "Is There a Religious Factor in Health Care Utilization?: A Review." *Social Science and Medicine* 27 (1988): 1369–79.

Spiegel, D., J. R. Bloom, H. C. Kraemer, and E. Gottheil. "Effect of Psychosocial Treatment on Survival of Patients with Metastatic Breast Cancer." *Lancet* 2 (1989): 888–91.

Wirth, D. P., J. T. Richardson, W. S. Eidelman, and A. C. O'Malley. "Full Thickness Dermal Wounds Treated with Non-Contact Therapeutic Touch: A Replication and Extension." *Complementary Therapies in Medicine* 1 (1993): 127–32.

CHAPTER 9

Wired for God

Armstrong, K. *A History of God: The 4,000-Year Quest of Judaism, Christianity and Islam.* New York: Knopf, 1993.

Begley, S. "Science of the Sacred." *Newsweek* (November 28, 1994): 56–59.

Benson, H., J. F. Beary, and M. P. Carol. "The Relaxation Response." *Psychiatry* 37 (1974): 37–46.

Blackmore, S. *Dying to Live: Near-Death Experiences.* Buffalo, NY: Prometheus Books, 1993.

Cummings, N. A., and G. R. VandenBos. "The Twenty Years Kaiser-Permanente Experience with Psychotherapy and Medical Utilization: Implications for National Health Policy and National Health Insurance." *Health Policy Quarterly* 1 (1981): 159–75.

Cytowic, R. E. *The Man Who Tasted Shapes: A Bizarre Medical Mystery Offers Revolutionary Insights into Emotions, Reasoning and Consciousness.* New York: G. P. Putnam, 1993.

Damasio, A. *Descartes' Error: Emotion, Reason and the Human Brain.* New York: Grosset/Putnam, 1994.

Gallup, G. H., Jr., and S. Jones. *100 Questions and Answers: Religion in America*. Princeton: Princeton Religion Research Center, 1989.

Harrison, K. "In His Brother's Shadow." *New York Times Book Review* (May 29, 1994): 3,12.

Holt, J. "At the Intersection of Science and Religion." *Wall Street Journal*, October 10, 1994.

Johnson, G. "Physicists Weigh In: The Quark Is a Porker." *New York Times*, March 5, 1995.

Johnson, S. As quoted in J. Bartlett. *Familiar Quotations*. Fourteenth Edition, E. M. Beck (ed.). Boston: Little, Brown, 1968.

Kantrowitz, B., P. King, D. Rosenberg, K. Springen, P. Wingert, T. Namuth, and T. T. Gegax. "In Search of the Sacred." *Newsweek* (November 28, 1994): 52–62.

Kolb, E. As quoted in S. Begley. "Science of the Sacred." *Newsweek* (November 28, 1994): 56.

Miles, J. *God: A Biography*. New York: Knopf, 1995.

Steinem, G. *Revolution from Within: A Book of Self-Esteem*. Boston: Little, Brown, 1992.

Templeton, J. W. (ed.). *Evidence of Purpose: Scientists Discover the Creator.* New York: Continuum, 1994.

Tipler, F. J. *The Physics of Immortality: Modern Cosmology, God and the Resurrection of the Dead*. New York: Doubleday, 1994.

CHAPTER 10
Optimal Medicine, Optimal Health

American Medical Association. *Physician Characteristics and Distribution in the U.S. 1994.* G. Roback, L. Randolph, B. Seidman, and T. Pasko (eds.). Chicago: Department of Data Services, 1994.

American Medical Association. *Physician Marketplace Statistics 1994.* M. L. Gonzalez (ed.). Chicago: Center for Health Policy Research, 1994.

Antoni, M. H., L. Baggett, G. Ironson, A. LaPerriere, S. August, N. Klimas, N. Schneiderman, and M. A. Fletcher. "Cognitive-Behavioral Stress Management Intervention Buffers Distress Responses and Immunologic Changes Following Notification of HIV-1 Seropositivity." *Journal of Consulting and Clinical Psychology* 59 (1991): 906–15.

Benson, H., and R. Friedman. "The Three-Legged Stool." *Mind/Body Medicine* 1 (1995): 1–2.

Benson, H., C. Kyle, and G. H. Gallup, Jr. (Unpublished Data).

Burton, R. *The Anatomy of Melancholy*. Oxford: John Lichfield and James Short. (1621). As quoted in T. A. Droege. *The Faith Factor in Healing*. Philadelphia: Trinity Press International, 1991.

Caudill, M., R. Schnable, P. C. Zuttermeister, H. Benson, and R. Friedman. "Decreased Clinic Utilization by Chronic Pain Patients: Response to Behavioral Medicine Intervention." *Clinical Journal of Pain* 7 (1991): 305–10.

Caudill, M. *Managing Pain Before It Manages You*. New York: Guilford, 1994.

Cummings, N. A., and G. R. VandenBos. "The Twenty Years Kaiser-Permanente Experience with Psychotherapy and Medical Utilization: Implications for National Health Policy and National Health Insurance." *Health Policy Quarterly* 1 (1981): 159–75.

Eisenberg, D. M., R. C. Kessler, C. Foster, F. E. Norlock, D. R. Calkins, and T. L. Delbanco. "Unconventional Medicine in the United States: Prevalence, Costs and Patterns of Use." *New England Journal of Medicine* 328 (1993): 246–52.

Fawzy, F. I., N. W. Fawzy, C. S. Hyun, R. Elashoff, D. Guthrie, J. L. Fahey, and D. L. Morton. "Malignant Melanoma: Effects of an Early Structured Psychiatric Intervention, Coping and Affective State on Recurrence and Survival 6 Years Later." *Archives of General Psychiatry* 50 (1993): 681–89.

Friedman, R., P. C. Zuttermeister, and H. Benson. "Unconventional Medicine [letter]." *New England Journal of Medicine* 329 (1993): 1201.

Hellman, C. J., M. Budd, J. Borysenko, D. C. McClelland, and H.

Benson. "A Study of the Effectiveness of Two Group Behavioral Medicine Interventions for Patients with Psychosomatic Complaints." *Behavioral Medicine* 16 (1990): 165–73.

Inui, T. S. As quoted in *The Economist* (December 10, 1994): 89–90.

Kennell, J., M. Klaus, S. McGrath, S. Robertson, and C. Hinkley. "Continuous Emotional Support During Labor in a U.S. Hospital: A Randomized Controlled Trial." *Journal of the American Medical Association* 265 (1991): 2197–2201.

Kroenke, K., and A. D. Mangelsdorff. "Common Symptoms in Ambulatory Care: Incidence, Evaluation, Therapy and Outcome." *American Journal of Medicine* 86 (1989): 262–66.

Lorig, K. R., P. D. Mazonson, and H. R. Holman. "Evidence Suggesting That Health Education for Self-Management in Patients with Chronic Arthritis Has Sustained Health Benefits While Reducing Health Care Costs." *Arthritis and Rheumatism* 36 (1993): 439–46.

Mumford, E., H. J. Schlesinger, and G. V. Glass. "The Effect of Psychological Intervention on Recovery from Surgery and Heart Attacks: An Analysis of the Literature." *American Journal of Public Health* 72 (1982): 141–51.

Ornish, D., S. E. Brown, L. W. Scherwitz, J. H. Billings, W. T. Armstrong, T. A. Ports, S. M. McLanahan, R. L. Kirkeeide, R. J. Brand, and K. L. Gould. "Can Lifestyle Changes Reverse Coronary Heart Disease? The Lifestyle Heart Trial." *Lancet* 336 (1990): 129–33.

Pallak, M. S., N. A. Cummings, H. Dorken, and C. J. Henke. "Effects of Mental Health Treatment on Medical Costs." *Mind/Body Medicine* 1 (1995): 7–12.

Robinson, J. S., M. L. Schwartz, K. S. Magwene, S. A. Krengel, and D. Tamburello. "The Impact of Fever Health Education on Clinic Utilization." *American Journal of Diseases of Children* 143 (1989): 698–704.

Sobel, D. "Mind Matters, Money Matters: The Cost-Effectiveness of Clinical Behavioral Medicine." *Mental Medicine Update* (1993): 1–8.

Sobel, D. "Mind/Body Medicine: Is It Really 'Alternative'?" *Mental Medicine Update* 4 (1995): 1–2.

U.S. Department of Health and Human Services. *Health*

United States 1993. Pub. No. (PHS) 94-1232. Hyattsville, MD: Public Health Service, 1994.

Wilson, S. R., P. Scamagas, D. F. German, G. W. Hughes, S. Lulla, S. Coss, L. Chardon, R. G. Thomas, N. Starr-Schneidkraut, and F. B. Stancavage. "A Controlled Trial of Two Forms of Self-Management Education for Adults with Asthma." *American Journal of Medicine* 94 (1993): 564–76.

CHAPTER 11
Trust Your Instincts, Trust Your Doctor

Ambady, N., and R. Rosenthal. "Half a Minute: Predicting Teacher Evaluations from Thin Slices of Nonverbal Behavior and Physical Attractiveness." *Journal of Personality and Social Psychology* 64 (1993): 431–41.

Bradsher, K. "As 1 Million Americans Leave Ranks of Insured, Debate Heats Up, Medicaid Battle Looms." *New York Times,* August 27, 1995, p. 1.

Holmes, O. W. *The Writings of Oliver Wendell Holmes.* Vol. 9, Medical Essays. Cambridge, MA: Riverside Press, 1891.

Letvak, R. "Putting the Placebo Effect into Practice." *Patient Care* 29 (1995): 93–102.

Peabody, F. W. *The Care of the Patient.* Cambridge, MA: Harvard University Press, 1927.

Raymond, A. G. *The HMO Health Care Companion: A Consumer's Guide to Managed Care Networks.* New York: HarperPerennial, 1994.

Shaw, G. B. *The Doctor's Dilemma.* Ayot St. Lawrence (ed.). New York: W.H. Wise, 1930.

"Why Doctors." *The Economist* (December 10, 1994): 89–90.

CHAPTER 12
The Ills of Information

Barinaga, M. "To Sleep, Perchance to . . . Learn? New Studies Say Yes." *Science* 265 (1994): 603–4.

Barsky, A. J. *Worried Sick: Our Troubled Quest for Wellness.* Boston: Little, Brown, 1988.

Becker, M. H. "The Tyranny of Health Promotion." *Public Health Reviews* 14 (1986): 15–25.

Benson, H. *Your Maximum Mind.* New York: Times Books/Random House, 1987.

Benson, H., and E. Stuart. *The Wellness Book: A Comprehensive Guide to Maintaining Health and Treating Stress-Related Illness.* New York: Fireside, 1993.

Champion, F. P., and R. Taylor. "Mass Hysteria Associated with Insect Bites." *Journal of the South Carolina Medical Association* 59 (1963): 351–53.

Davidson, A. "Choreomania: A Historical Sketch with Some Account of an Epidemic Observed in Madagascar." *Edinburgh Medical Journal* 13 (1867): 124–36.

Davy, R. D. "St. Vitus' Dance and Kindred Affectations." *The Cincinnati Lancet and Clinic* 4 (1880): 440–45.

DeAngelis, B. *Real Moments.* New York: Delacorte, 1994.

Frankel, F. H. "Discovering New Memories in Psychotherapy—Childhood Revisited, Fantasy or Both?" *New England Journal of Medicine* 333 (1995): 591–94.

Freidson, E. *Profession of Medicine: A Study of the Sociology of Applied Knowledge.* New York: Dodd, Mead, 1970.

Hannay, D. R. *The Symptom Iceberg: A Study of Community Health.* London, Boston: Routledge & Kegan Paul, 1979.

Inlander, C. B., L. S. Levin, and E. Weiner. *Medicine on Trial: The Appalling Story of Ineptitude, Malfeasance, Neglect and Arrogance.* New York: Prentice-Hall, 1988.

Kabat-Zinn, J. *Full Catastrophe Living: Using the Wisdom of Your Body and Mind to Face Stress, Pain and Illness.* New York: Delacorte, 1990.

Mack, J. E. *Abduction: Human Encounters with Aliens.* New York: Scribner, 1994.

Martin, A. "History of the Dancing Mania: A Contribution to the Study of Psychic Mass Infection." *American Journal of Clinical Medicine* 30 (1923): 265–71.

McLeod, W. R. "Merphos Poisoning or Mass Panic?" *Australian and New Zealand Journal of Psychiatry* 9 (1975): 225–29.

Meichenbaum, D. *Cognitive-Behavior Modification: An Integrative Approach.* New York: Plenum, 1977.

Milton, J. *Paradise Lost.* London: 1946.

Morrison, T. *Song of Solomon.* New York: Knopf, 1977.

Myers, L. "Many Kids Scared of Future; Even Good Parents at a Loss to Deal with It." *San Diego Union-Tribune,* May 11, 1995, p. A7.

Ofshe, R., and E. Watters. *Making Monsters: False Memories, Psychotherapy and Sexual Hysteria.* New York: Scribner, 1994.

Rosen, G. "Psychopathology in the Social Process: Dance Frenzies, Demonic Possession, Revival Movements and Similar So-Called Psychic Epidemics." *Bulletin of Historical Medicine* 36 (1962): 13–44.

Rosenthal, E. "Maybe You're Sick, Maybe We Can Help." *New York Times,* April 11, 1994.

Rubenstein, C. "Wellness Is All." *Psychology Today* (1982): 28–37.

Shorter, E. *Bedside Manners: The Troubled History of Doctors and Patients.* New York: Simon & Schuster, 1985.

Small, G. W., and A. M. Nicholi, Jr. "Mass Hysteria Among Schoolchildren: Early Loss As a Predisposing Factor." *Archives of General Psychiatry* 39 (1982): 721–24.

Steinberg, D. "Personal Best." *GQ* (February 1995): 108.

Suib-Cohen, S. *Secrets of a Very Good Marriage: Lessons from the Sea.* New York: Crown, 1993.

Vaillant, G. E. *Adaptation to Life.* Boston: Little, Brown, 1977.

Vrazo, F. "They Blame Themselves for Breast Cancer: Still Unknown Cause, Yet Some Feel Guilty." *San Diego Union-Tribune,* October 31, 1994, p. B-3.

CHAPTER 13

Timeless Healing

St. Anselm. "Proslogion. Chap 3." As quoted in J. Bartlett. *Familiar Quotations.* Fourteenth Edition, E. M. Beck (ed.). Boston: Little, Brown, 1968.

Armstrong, K. *A History of God: The 4,000-Year Quest of Judaism, Christianity and Islam.* New York: Knopf, 1993.

Benson, H., A. Kornhaber, C. Kornhaber, M. N. LeChanu, P. C. Zuttermeister, P. Myers, and R. Friedman. "Increases in Positive Psychological Characteristics with a New Relaxation-Response Curriculum in High School Students." *Journal for Research and Development in Education* 27 (1994): 226–31.

Cytowic, R. E. *The Man Who Tasted Shapes: A Bizarre Medical Mystery Offers Revolutionary Insights into Emotions, Reasoning and Consciousness.* New York: G.P. Putnam, 1993.

Dunkin, A. "Meditation, The New Balm for Corporate Stress." *Business Week* (May 10, 1993): 86–87.

Heraclitus. As quoted in J. Bartlett. *Familiar Quotations.* Fourteenth Edition, E. M. Beck (ed.). Boston: Little, Brown, 1968, p. 77.

The Holy Bible: Old and New Testaments in the King James Version. Nashville, TN: Nelson, 1983.

James, W. "Pragmatism: Lecture 1. 1907." As quoted in J. Bartlett. *Familiar Quotations.* Fourteenth Edition, E. M. Beck (ed.). Boston: Little, Brown, 1968.

Niebuhr, R. As quoted in J. Bartlett. *Familiar Quotations.* Fourteenth Edition, E. M. Beck (ed.). Boston: Little, Brown, 1968.

Ornish, D., S. E. Brown, L. W. Scherwitz, J. H. Billings, W. T. Armstrong, T. A. Ports, S. M. McLanahan, R. L. Kirkeeide, R. J. Brand, and K. L. Gould. "Can Lifestyle Changes Reverse Coronary Heart Disease? The Lifestyle Heart Trial." *Lancet* 336 (1990): 129–33.

Stratford, S. "Leaders Learn to Heed the Voice Within." *Fortune* (August 22, 1994): 92–100.

INDEX

psychosomatic
nocebo effect
anniversary reaction
prerogative
synesthesia   escalating
at bay   jaundice
  abasement   relaxation response
                                monkey mind
tsog tsuam   (stuff of life)
SUNDS   flabbergasted
  exacerbated
ventricular fibrillation

TEXT PERMISSIONS